Violence and Aggression in the Workplace

A practical guide for all healthcare staff

Paul Linsley

Senior Lecturer in Nursing
The Faculty of Health, Life and Social Sciences
The University of Lincoln

Foreword by

Professor Dame June Clark

Radcliffe Publishing
Oxford ● Seattle

Radcliffe Publishing Ltd
18 Marcham Road
Abingdon
Oxon OX14 1AA
United Kingdom

www.radcliffe-oxford.com
Electronic catalogue and worldwide online ordering facility.

British Library Cataloguing in Publication Data

A catalogue record for this book is available from the British Library.

ISBN-10: 1 85775 784 X
ISBN-13: 978 1 85775 784 2

Typeset by Aarontype Ltd, Easton, Bristol
Printed and bound by TJ International Ltd, Padstow, Cornwall

Contents

Foreword

The first time it happened to me I was stunned. It was just so unexpected. I was a newly qualified health visitor, working in a 'nice', middle class area, visiting a 'nice' family with a new baby in the middle of a Monday morning. I didn't expect the 'eyeball to eyeball' tirade from the smartly dressed father about how health visitors were nosey government spies and anyone who worked in the public sector was a lousy parasite on the nation's economy. I wasn't physically hurt, but I was certainly shaken, and it affected my practice as a health visitor for quite a long time.

So I was delighted to read this book, and I commend it to you. In those days violence and aggression were expected only by those working in acute psychiatric settings, or big city accident and emergency departments, or as community nurses in 'tough' areas. Nowadays we know it can happen to any health worker, any place, any time, and all of us need, like the boy scouts, to 'be prepared'.

This is not a book to be carried around in the back pocket and whipped out in an emergency. It ought to be read by everyone during their initial preparation, used during CPD and in-service education, and kept handy for reference. I would have also found it helpful to read afterwards, to help me better understand what had happened and why, and to come to terms with it.

Professor Dame June Clark DBE PhD RN RHV FRCN
Professor Emeritus
University of Wales Swansea
May 2006

Preface

The following book is aimed at all healthcare staff that may have cause to come into contact with the patient or their family, including reception staff and those that deal with complaints. It is designed to reflect good practice which is in use throughout the NHS and other organisations to help protect healthcare staff from the risk that is violence and aggression. While the book aims to be as comprehensive as possible, such work cannot cater for every situation that may or may not occur within a working environment. As such the book should be used as a reference source and general guide only. Specific interventions and procedures will be provided by individual employers, and these should be adhered to in the event of an incident occurring.

The author has been keen to avoid the word victim, as this implies a degree of helplessness, and would instead ask the reader to replace this with the word target, as this better describes the role in which the individuals find themselves as part of the assault process. Within each chapter there are a number of different types of information and activities that are highlighted within the text. This includes keywords and concepts to help structure thinking and understanding around the topic.

Paul Linsley
May 2006

About the author

Paul began his career as a general nurse working within acute medicine. Following conversion to mental health nursing he gained valuable experience in a variety of clinical settings, and is a nurse specialist within acute mental health care. He has held a number of managerial and educational posts, teaching on a number of courses for the University of Nottingham, and now works for the University of Lincoln as a Senior Lecturer in Nursing. In addition to this Paul sits on a number of national forums for the Royal College of Nursing as well as being a nurse advisor to the Department of Health. He has had a number of articles published and is actively involved in the research of violence and aggression within the healthcare setting.

Chapter 7 of this book was written by Julie Dixon who is a health lecturer with the University of Nottingham, teaching mental health and gender theory. She works within a life-course perspective, and her current research and interests focus around women as recipients and providers of healthcare, particularly with regards to those suffering from a mental disorder. She teaches on a number of modules that explore the relationships between gender, the family and health, as well as being involved in a number of outside agencies seeking to promote equality within healthcare service provision.

Acknowledgements

Thanks to Vicki, Andrew and Adel for their continued love and support. Thanks also to Rodney, Andy and Carol for their friendship and encouragement. I would also like to acknowledge the help of Julie and Jan in putting this book together.

Chapter 1

Violence and aggression

Introduction

The level of violence and aggression against healthcare staff has become an important issue in recent years.[1] Indicators would suggest that anyone who works for the health and social care sector and who has contact with the general public is at risk from such behaviour.[2] This is not a new problem and reflects wider concerns about violent crime in society generally. More and more healthcare staff face the prospect of violence and aggression in the workplace, not only from the people that they care for, but from strangers and within families.[3]

People who behave in ways that bring them into conflict with others make special demands on a service and its staff who are already under pressure.[4] Violence and aggression raise special concern because they significantly increase the risk of injury and harm. This can have an impact on staff confidence and morale as well as patient care. Threats, aggravation and tension caused by potential aggressors can lead to stress-related problems, emotional burnout and result in some staff leaving the service altogether.[5]

Appropriate interventions from healthcare staff are crucial to the immediate physical and psychological safety of themselves and those that they care for.[6] As with other risks, reducing violence and aggression requires a systematic approach involving a number of strategies. Measures to reduce violence and aggression need to be based on sound risk assessment and risk management, underpinned by effective strategies worked out in collaboration with other agencies such as the local police department and prosecution service.[7]

Defining violence and aggression

One of the difficulties in addressing violence and aggression is that they are not easy to define.[3] Violence and aggression are subjective terms that mean different things to different people and groups. This means that the same kind of violent incident may have quite different impacts according to the individual involved. Because of this, healthcare organisations and staff groups have defined violence and aggression in different ways for different purposes. However, in order to recognise, address, and prevent violence and aggression, healthcare staff must have a clear understanding as to what these terms mean. This requires a description that encompasses the different forms that violence and aggression can take, while allowing for personal interpretation and understanding. In doing this, it allows staff to take ownership of the problem and goes some way to acknowledging their concerns.

The Department of Health has defined violence and aggression as being:

> Any incident where staff are abused, threatened or assaulted in circumstances relating to their work, involving an explicit or implicit challenge to their safety, well being or health.[8]

This is similar to the definition used by the Health Development Agency, which is as follows:

> Any incident in which a person working in the healthcare sector is verbally abused, threatened or assaulted by a patient or member of the public in circumstances relating to his or her employment.[4]

The two definitions reflect the fact that violence is not restricted to acts of aggression that may result in physical harm but incorporates behaviour, including the use of gestures and language, that may cause the subject to become afraid or feel threatened and abused. Threats may be perceived or real, and there does not have to be physical injury for the violence to be a workplace hazard.

In a further definition, the International Labour Organisation defines violence at work as being:

> All forms of behaviour which produce damaging or hurtful effects, physically or emotionally to staff in the course of their work.[7]

This definition suggests that harm could be caused unintentionally. This could occur with certain cultural differences as much as personal preferences in the way in which staff members or the public wish to be treated.

Lastly the Counter Fraud and Security Management Service (CFSMS), a special health authority within the NHS, who have overall responsibility for the management of violence and aggression within the healthcare sector, use the following definition:

> The intentional application of force to the person, without lawful justification, resulting in physical injury or personal discomfort.[9]

This, however, fails to take into account unintentional violence which may be the result of a patient having received a head injury following a road traffic accident.

Whatever definition is eventually decided upon should have meaning for those that are going to use it, and ensure recognition of the problem. Promoting the issue of violence and aggression within the healthcare setting is as important as defining it, if not more so.

The different forms that aggression can take

Whatever definition is used, it is clear that in a working-life context violence and aggression vary considerably. It is therefore useful to consider the various forms these can take.

In general terms, aggressive or violent acts can be seen as being:

- uncivil behaviour: lack of respect for others
- physical or verbal aggression: intention to injure
- assault: intention to harm another person.[5]

Buss offers the following classification system in which he describes aggression as a mixture of physical/verbal; active/passive; or direct/indirect:[10]

- *physical/active/direct*: one-off, acute incidents that usually include physical violence, for instance, a drunken fight, a mugging, a confused patient lashing out, or routine and chronic incidents, such as being physically or sexually abused or bullied
- *physical/active/indirect*: persuading someone else to do harm, such as advocating smacking as a form of discipline
- *physical/passive/direct*: physically preventing someone from attaining a desired goal, such as a senior colleague deliberately blocking access to a post
- *physical/passive/indirect*: refusing to perform necessary tasks
- *verbal/active/direct*: using insults or being derogatory about another person, for example being sworn at, or made the target of racial or sexual abuse
- *verbal/active/indirect*: spreading malicious gossip about others or undermining confidence by belittling their capabilities and appearance
- *verbal/passive/direct*: refusing to speak or answer questions
- *verbal/passive/indirect*: failing to take responsibility for contributing vocally, such as not speaking up in another's defence when he or she is unfairly criticised.

Using this framework, aggression can be seen as being any form of behaviour used with the intention to harm or injure another person. However, as has already been pointed out, acts of aggression can also be unintentional in nature. In addition to this, acts of aggression can be directed either outwardly towards others or inwardly at the individual, for example self-harm. Property damage is also a form of violence. While it may not threaten the safety of staff it can be stressful and distressing to witness. Consequently, aggressive acts can be seen as existing on a continuum from verbal or emotional acts to serious physical harm (*see* Figure 1.1).[11]

It is also important to recognise at this point that aggressive acts can be enacted in writing, via email and over the phone, allowing greater access to staff than ever before.

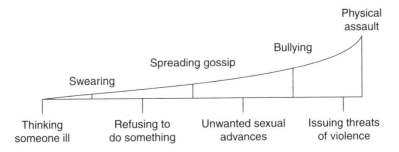

Figure 1.1 Escalating aggression.

Activity 1.1

What do the terms violence and aggression mean to you? Reflect on any incidents from your work. What types of aggression have you experienced and which of these have you found most distressing and why?

Box 1.1 lists other words associated with healthcare violence and aggression.

Box 1.1 Other words associated with healthcare violence and aggression, and their definitions[12–14]

- *Assault*: a violent attack; an unlawful physical attack upon another; an attempt or offer to do violence to another, with or without battery.
- *Battery*: an assault with actual touching or other violence upon another.
- *Controlling behaviour*: preventing someone by force from acting freely. This can include keeping them from seeing relatives and friends, not letting them have a job or not letting them spend money or have access to their personal belongings.
- *Emotional abuse*: saying things on purpose to frighten the other person or putting them down to make them feel bad.
- *Harassment*: any action, whether verbal or physical, single or repeated, deliberate or unintentional that is unwanted or unwelcome.
- *Psychological violence*: intentional use of power against another person or group that can result in harm to physical, mental, spiritual, moral or social development.
- *Physical violence*: the use of physical force against another person or group that results in physical, sexual, or psychological harm.
- *Sexual abuse*: forcing or encouraging someone to take part in sexual behaviour in any way that makes them uncomfortable.
- *Sexual harassment*: any objectionable, unwanted, or unwelcome attention to a person because of his or her sex.
- *Threat*: a declaration of an intention or determination to inflict punishment, injury, death, or loss on someone in retaliation for, or conditionally upon, some action or course.

Classification of the assailant

As well as a definition to describe incidents there also needs to be an agreed framework to describe assailants. This information is useful in the monitoring and planning of services in response to risk. Wykes provided the following framework by which to do this:

- *direct user of the service*: where the assailant is in current receipt of a service provided by the healthcare worker [own words] at the time of the incident, i.e. the assailant could be described as a patient, client or user

- *indirect user of the service*: where the assailant is closely associated with a current user (relative, friend, etc) of the service
- *no current user of the service*: where the assailant does not receive the healthcare service and is not closely associated with a user of the service.[13]

In describing assailants in this way there is a recognition that violence and aggression occur not only as a result of the service provided, but by association with it and in absence of user involvement. This is similar to the much-adopted classification scheme proposed by the Occupational Safety and Health Administration:[14]

- *type I*: where the assailant has no legitimate relationship to the workplace and the main object of the attack is cash or some other valuable commodity
- *type II*: which involve some form of assault by a person who is either the recipient or the object of a service provided by the affected workplace or the victim
- *type III*: where another employee, a supervisor, or an acquaintance of the worker perpetrates an assault.

Viitasara and Ohon have argued that there is a fourth type of violence that arises out of wider social and economic pressures, for example an increased demand on healthcare services and provision in times of financial hardship might lead to staff adopting more controlling methods to manage aggression, because of demands on limited resources.[15,16]

Aggression within healthcare

Healthcare staff are faced with dealing with people who are often in desperate need of attention and care, which they may, through ill-health, age or other circumstances, be unable to provide for themselves. They work with people from across the whole of society, in circumstances that may be difficult and demanding. Patients may be anxious and worried about coming into hospital and what might happen to them. Some patients may be predisposed towards violence and aggression as a means of coping.[17] Likewise, it may be that the patient's relatives or friends express their frustrations or distress through aggression towards staff. While these factors do not excuse acts of aggression, it is easy to understand why healthcare staff and those that they care for occasionally come into conflict. It is important to recognise at this point that aggression is very rarely purposeless. People are aggressive either because they want something to happen or because they want something to stop happening. In clinical settings, aggression and violence may be used by patients as a way of getting what they want. Violent acts may be used to force change or to regain or maintain control. Rewards from violence include attention from staff, and status and prestige among the patient group.[18] For example, the patient who behaves violently is observed more frequently and has more opportunities to discuss concerns with their doctor and nursing staff. This situation is likely to test the healthcare worker's ability to cope with the psychological consequences of threats and assaults even further, and in a way the cycle becomes self-perpetuating.[19]

Aggressive actions can also originate from colleagues.[20–22] Many tensions can occur within work teams, and in healthy organisational cultures, those tensions can be a valuable force for initiating change.[20] Psychological violence is often perpetrated through repeated behaviour, of a type which may alone be relatively minor but which cumulatively can become a very serious form of violence. Although a single incident can suffice, psychological violence often consists of repeated, unwelcome, unreciprocated, and imposed actions, which may have a devastating effect on their target. This is typical in bullying and harassment, which are perpetrated through repeated or persistent behaviour.[16] Bullying turns to harassment when it is targeted repeatedly toward the same person or staff group and the chosen target is to some extent defenceless in the face of the perpetrator.[23] These persistently negative attacks on their personal and professional performance are typically unpredictable, irrational and unfair.

Bullying is a real problem within the health service, causing many staff to take sickness absence or early retirement and to leave the service altogether.[16] Most organisations now have polices and procedures for dealing with bullying and harassment that outline what is and what is not acceptable behaviour. Penalties for transgression can result in dismissal. However, proving someone has been a bully is difficult, particularly if it has been done in a covert way (*see* Box 1.2).

Box 1.2 Recognising bullying in the workplace[22]

- Making life difficult for those who have the potential to do the bully's job better than the bully
- Punishing others for being too competent, by constant criticism or by removing their responsibilities, often giving them trivial tasks to do instead
- Refusing to delegate because they feel they cannot trust anyone else
- Shouting at staff to get things done
- Persistently picking on people in front of others, or in private
- Insisting that a way of doing things is always right
- Keeping individuals in their place, blocking their promotion
- If someone challenges a bully's authority, overloading them with work and reducing the deadlines, hoping that they will fail at what they do
- Feeling envious of another's professional or social ability, so setting out to make them appear incompetent, or make their lives miserable, in the hope of getting them dismissed or making them resign

---

The incidence of violence and aggression in the healthcare setting

The true incidence of workplace violence in the healthcare setting is difficult to estimate. Differences in definitions of workplace violence and aggression, the scope of the healthcare industry and significant under-reporting of violent incidents by healthcare workers make compilations of data regarding the prevalence of violence near impossible.

However, statistical indicators would suggest that violence and aggression in the healthcare setting are on the increase, and that all staff that have direct contact with patients and their relatives are vulnerable, including reception staff and those who have to deal with complaints. Whittington has argued that the increase in reported incidents can be attributed to a decreased tolerance of violence on the part of healthcare staff, and an increased fear of experiencing it.[24] It has also been argued that some of the increase in violence and aggression can be attributed to the unrealistic public expectations of what health services can provide.[25] Wells and Bowers describe how inadequate staffing levels, increasing workloads, and the near-indifference to the welfare needs of healthcare workers have helped create conditions where aggression can flourish.[26] While emergency departments and psychiatric settings still continue to be the focus of much attention with regard to workplace violence, the rationalisation of healthcare services in recent years has led to large numbers of disgruntled clients, and the advent of care in the community programmes with their consequent early discharge from healthcare agencies, has resulted in an increased risk of violence across many healthcare settings. How much of this increase is the result of better reporting mechanisms within the NHS and a heightened awareness amongst staff that such behaviour need not be tolerated is unclear.[27]

In 2000, the Department of Health conducted a national survey into the reported incidences of violence and aggression in NHS trusts and authorities in England.[28] A total of 84 273 violent or abusive incidents were reported. This was an increase of some 24 000 over the previous year 1998–99 (the only other occasion on which this sort of information had been collected on a national basis). In 2001 they conducted a follow-up survey which showed a further 13% increase to 95 501 reported incidents. Reasons given for the increase included better awareness of reporting, increased hospital activity, higher patient expectations, and frustrations due to increased waiting times.[29] In 2002–2003, the number had again risen to 116 000.[25] Within this study the average number of incidents for NHS mental health and learning disability trusts was reported as being almost two and a half times the average for all trusts, despite evidence that staff working in mental health units were much less likely to report verbal abuse.

In 2004, the Commission for Health Improvement conducted a survey of healthcare staff of which 203 911 responded.[30] Findings showed that 15% of respondents had experienced physical violence at work in the previous year – usually from patients or their relatives – and 37% had experienced harassment, bullying or abuse.

In the absence of healthcare research, many campaigns use data gained from crime surveys. The 2000 British Crime Survey showed that just under half (46%) of assaults at work resulted in some type of injury, primarily bruising and black eyes.[31] However, 1% of the injuries resulted in broken bones. Workplace violence also has an emotional impact on victims. Seven out of ten victims of workplace assault, and nearly three out of four victims of workplace violence and threat reported being affected emotionally. While actual physical assaults can and do take place in healthcare settings, verbal aggression and threats of violence remain the most common.[28–30] Whatever its exact form, however, the fact remains that healthcare workers are disproportionately at risk of workplace violence when compared with other workforce sectors.[16,32,33] Yet despite the risks and legal obligations, few hospitals are known to have explicit strategies to deal with the potential threat to their employees.[34]

Although there is a high risk of workplace violence across all healthcare occupations, most indicators suggest that it is the nursing profession that is most at risk, closely followed by ambulance and medical staff.[28-30] In a survey of health-care personnel across all departments of a general hospital, Whittington *et al.* found that 21% had been physically assaulted over a one-year period, and nurses at all levels were more likely to be assaulted than any other occupational group.[35] The British Crime Survey showed that female nurses had at least four times the average risk of job-related violence and threats when compared with the average rate across all occupations.[33] A systematic review of the literature on violence against nurses in the UK revealed that a minimum of 9.5% of general hospital nurses were subjected to physical assault (with or without injury) in any one year.[26]

Box 1.3   Occupations at risk from violence and aggression[25,28,31]

(Note that health and community services head the list)

- *Health and community services*: nurses, doctors, ambulance officers, cashiers, welfare workers, ward helpers, accommodation services workers
- *Government, administration and education*: police, prison and other government enforcement officers, school teachers, probation officers, collection agency workers
- *Business services*: finance sector, counter staff managers
- *Transport and storage*: guards, bus drivers, taxi drivers, and couriers
- *Retail trade*: all sales and support staff
- *Consumer services*: hospitality staff, managers, administration and other occupations

---

Collectively these surveys were able to demonstrate that the number of violent incidents varied by trust type. They were also able to demonstrate the differences in the way that trusts collected data on violent incidents. For example, the definition in one trust might include verbal abuse, and in another trust it might be excluded. Most importantly the surveys found that there was a significant under-reporting of violence directed at staff working in the NHS, and that this was historical. Under-reporting of the occurrence of violence and aggression has been attributed to the absence of formal channels designed to record this information, lack of time, reluctance to fill in forms, fear of being blamed, embarrassment and an acceptance of violence and aggression as part of the job, while others fear that flak from patients reflects their professional failure to manage challenging situations appropriately.[28-30] Others do not report incidents simply because they do not believe that anything will come of it, either in terms of prosecution or feedback from their employer, and therefore feel reporting is a waste of time. Failure to address under-reporting of incidents is a major concern because it means that available data are incomplete, and strategies implemented to reduce violence will only be partially successful.[36]

The effects of violence and aggression on staff

The consequences of violence and aggression on the wellbeing of staff are increasingly well documented.[25,29,37] A number of factors appear to influence the extent and severity of the effects of violence and aggression, such as the sex, age and experience of the person attacked. Staff who are victims of violence tend to distance themselves from patients.[38] They may experience recurrent depression and anxiety, guilt and self-doubt, feelings of powerlessness and low self-esteem.[7,26] Emotional reactions can take the form of rage, anxiety, a sense of helplessness, irritation, fear of returning to the location of the incident, and feelings and thoughts that something should have been done to prevent what happened. Reactions such as anger, disappointment, shock and ambivalence have also been reported. A survey of members of the Royal College of Nursing showed that nurses who were assaulted had poorer psychological wellbeing than those that were not assaulted.[20] They were also twice as likely to have acute psychological problems, with frequently assaulted individuals most affected. There is also the possibility that exposure to violence and aggression could lead to an increased risk of post-traumatic stress disorder (PTSD), psychological burnout or other stress reactions. The reaction of individuals usually depends on the nature of the incident, the person's own experiences, skills and personality, and the extent to which they were directly or indirectly involved.

Exposure to physical violence is also associated with behavioural reactions and change, such as social withdrawal. This may affect social relationships at work, as well as relationships outside of work.[16] Those frequently exposed to violence at work have higher rates of absenteeism and provide a lower standard of care than those who are not exposed.[28] Marital problems and inability to become involved in social activity are not uncommon.[16]

In addition to the above, a substantially higher number of people worry about threats and physical assaults than those that actually experience violence and aggression at work. In some cases, worrying about violence and aggression represents a health risk.[28,29] Violence and aggression also have ramifications beyond those directly involved. Research has shown that witnessing violence and aggression may lead to fear of violent incidents, and as such has similar negative effects to being personally assaulted or attacked.[32]

While persistent abuse may be assumed to have a detrimental effect on staff, it is difficult to quantify the emotional distress caused by violence and aggression in the workplace. A number of research studies have demonstrated clear links between violence and aggression and staff sickness absence, turnover, lost productivity, and financial burden (*see* Box 1.4).[39] In some instances work may stop altogether and some workers may not be able to return to work for quite a period of time. International research aimed at estimating the cost of workplace violence and stress concluded that there are too many uncertainties and factors to consider, such as being able to identify the reasons for staff absences, to attempt detailed cost calculations; however it is estimated that violence and aggression accounts for millions of pounds in lost revenue each year.

Box 1.4   Effects of violence in the workplace[39]

- Higher incidence of patient complaints
- Higher risk of violent incidents
- Increased recruitment and retention costs

- Increased staff absence, reduced efficiency and performance at work
- Increased staff turnover
- Lowered reputation of the organisation
- Reduced staff morale
- Reduced staff numbers

Impact factors

A number of factors have been identified that, while they do not cause violence and aggression directly, do however have an impact on it and can enhance its effects.[40–42] Environmental factors, such as poor lighting, poor security, and accessibility of objects that can be used as weapons can increase the risk of violence. General discomfort such as being kept waiting in a crowed room can also cause anger and upset. Medical conditions or the influence of alcohol or drugs can exacerbate out of all proportion potentially minor irritants that would normally cause only slight upset or frustration.

Work-related characteristics, such as type of care setting (care home or hospital), form of employment (full-time or part-time working), working hours (day or night), work conditions (e.g. frequency of contact with care recipients, working in the homes of clients, working alone), work activities/tasks, organisational change (e.g. downsizing), and workload have also been studied, and are factors that may increase or decrease exposure and risk to healthcare violence and aggression.[43–45]

Understaffing may increase the risk of violence due to longer patient wait times, as can workers being left alone with patients. Workplace stressors, such as low supervisor support, work overload, poor workgroup relationships, or impending workplace changes, such as downsizing or restructuring, may also increase the risk of aggression in the workplace.[44]

In addition, recently employed staff have been found to be more at risk when compared with their more experienced colleagues.[46] By the same token, the presence of inexperienced staff and untrained staff can provide the opportunity for those that use violence and aggression as a coping strategy to engage in it. Similarly ward overcrowding is likely to contribute to increased violence by increasing patient arousal, impacting negatively on the perceived quality of patient care and increasing the opportunity for patient grievances with staff and patients.[47] Box 1.5 summarises the factors associated with increased risk of violence and aggression.

Box 1.5 Factors associated with increase risk of violence and aggression[7,12,15]

- Working in contact with the public
- Working with valuables and cash handling
- Working with people in distress
- Job insecurity

- Criminal activity
- Mental instability
- The influence of alcohol or other drugs
- Expression of irritation or frustration, such as dissatisfaction with poor service
- Feeling aggrieved due to unfair treatment, whether real or imagined
- Uncomfortable physical conditions
- Feelings of loss of control
- Geographical location, whether urban or rural, local crime rate and risk

The increased use of agency staff also has the potential to create an unfavourable working climate, affecting morale for the regular staff and patients. It has been suggested that when new personnel are appearing on a daily basis on the ward, there can be a reduction in continuity of care and this is particularly difficult and confusing situation for patients who are less able to develop relationships and interact with new people.

Healthcare settings are embedded in communities, which may influence the type and level of workplace violence experienced. High levels of violent crime or gang activity within a community, low levels of community resources, and mistrust or miscommunication between minority residents and majority providers may contribute to violence in the healthcare setting.[44,45] Larger societal factors, such as changing societal norms around the acceptance of aggression may have an impact on the risk of workplace violence. For example, there is the growing perception that acts of aggression within healthcare reflect similar findings within society, and that people are much more ready to resort to such behaviour as a means of coping and getting what they want.

Finally, a number of studies have attempted to explore the influences of race, culture, economics, and environmental factors on violent behaviour, all of which have been shown to have an impact on violence and aggression. Cultural norms help define acceptable and unacceptable behaviour and means of expressing feelings. Sanctions are applied to those who violate these norms through the legal system. By this means, society controls violent behaviour and attempts to maintain a safe existence for its members.[48] Unfortunately, this prohibition against violent behaviour may be extended to include any expression of anger. This can inhibit people from the healthy expression of angry feelings, and lead to other maladaptive responses, such as excessive drinking of alcohol.

A situational analysis of violence and aggression (taking into account the factors discussed) (*see* Figure 1.2) illustrates the complex nature of such acts and the many factors inherent therein. Applied to the workplace, aggression and violence are seen as a possible outcome of negative interpersonal interactions, which are, in turn, embedded in the broader social and organisational context in which they occur.

The model shown in Figure 1.2 illustrates the fact that not all forms of violence are identical in their social and psychological underpinnings; rather, a number of types of work-related violence can be distinguished and identified. This helps our understanding of the problem, and encourages us to think more widely about

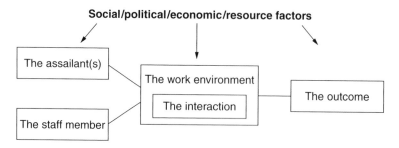

Figure 1.2 Violence in the workplace.

the issues involved. When the explanatory focus shifts from the individual to the situation, it is clear to see how organisational and sociopolitical factors come to be related to the incidents of violence and aggression.

In some cases, the particular job might include multiple risk situations. Social workers provide an example of an occupation in which organisational, social and political factors can be found, including:

- allocation of scarce resources
- compulsory admission of some mentally ill and mentally impaired people to hospital
- removal of children from some homes against the wishes of the parents
- investigation of cases of non-accidental injury to children
- compulsory removal of some elderly people from home to hospital
- supervision in the community of men and women with a history of potential or actual violence, some with an associated mental disorder.[49]

Violence and aggression then result as much from the characteristics of the healthcare worker and the organisation in which they work as it does from the characteristics of the individual service user.

Activity 1.2

Having read Chapter 1, have your ideas changed regarding violence and aggression? How have they changed, if at all? Compare your response with that of Activity 1.1.

References

1 Krug EG, Dahlberg LL, Mercy JA *et al.* (eds). *World Report on Violence and Health.* Geneva: World Health Organization; 2002.

2 Department of Health. *2000/2001 Survey of Reported Violent or Abusive Incidents, Accidents Involving Staff and Sickness Absence in NHS Authorities, in England.* London: Department of Health; 2001.

3 Royal College of Nursing. *Dealing with Violence against Nursing Staff: an RCN guide for nurses and managers.* London: Royal College of Nursing; 2003.

4 NHS Health Development Agency. *Violence and Aggression in General Practice: Guidance on assessment and management.* London: Department of Health; 2002.

5   European Agency for Safety and Health at Work (EASHW). *Violence at Work: Fact Sheet 24*. Brussels: European Agency for Safety and Health at Work; 2002.

6   Leather P, Brady C, Lawrence C *et al*. (eds). *Work-related Violence. Assessment and intervention*. London: Routledge; 1999.

7   Chappell D, Di Martino V. *Violence at Work* (2e). Geneva: International Labour Organisation; 2000.

8   Department of Health. *Campaign to Stop Violence against Staff Working in the NHS: NHS Zero Tolerance Zone*. Health Service Circular 1999/266. London: Department of Health.

9   Counter Fraud and Security Management Service. Conflict resolution training: implementing the national syllabus, 2003. In: Ferns T and Chojnacka I. Reporting incidents of violence and aggression towards NHS staff. *Nursing Standard*. 2005; **19**: 51–6.

10 Buss AH. *Personality: temperament, social behaviour and the self*. Boston: Allyn and Bacon; 1995.

11 Shepherd J (ed). *Violence in Health Care: a practical guide to coping with violence and caring for victims*. Oxford: Oxford University Press; 1994.

12 Di Martino V, Hoel H and Cooper CL. *Preventing Violence and Harassment in the Workplace*. Dublin: European Foundation for the Improvement of Living and Working Conditions; 2003.

13 Wykes T (ed.). *Violence and Health Care Professionals*. London: Chapman and Hall; 1994.

14 Occupational Safety and Health Administration. *Guidelines for Preventing Workplace Violence for Health and Social Service Workers*. Washington, DC: Occupational Safety and Health Administration; 1998.

15 Viitasara E. *Violence in Caring*. Stockholm: National Institute for Working Life; 2004.

16 Ohon N. Workplace violence: theories of causation and prevention strategies. *Journal of the American Association of Occupational Health Nurses*. 1994; **4**: 477–82.

17 Lindow V and McGeorge M. *Research Review on Violence Against Staff in Mental Health Community Settings*. London: Royal College of Psychiatry Research Unit; 2000.

18 Turnbull J and Paterson B. *Aggression and Violence: approaches to effective management*. London: MacMillan; 1999.

19 Burton R. Violence and aggression in the workplace. *Mental Health Care*. 1998; **2**: 105–108.

20 Royal College of Nursing. *Challenging Harassment and Bullying: guidance for RCN representatives, stewards and officers*. London: Royal College of Nursing; 2001.

21 Geddes D and Baron R. Workplace aggression as a consequence of negative feedback. *Management Communication Quarterly*. 1997; **10**: 433–55.

22 UNISON. *Guidance on Bullying*. London: UNISON; 1996.

23 Leymann H. The content and development of mobbing at work. *European Journal of Work and Organisational Psychology*. 1996; **5**: 165–84.

24 Whittington R. Violence to nurses: prevalence and risk factors. *Nursing Standard*. 1997; **12**: 49–56.

25 Health Services Commission. *A Safer Place to Work: protecting NHS hospital and ambulance staff from violence and aggression*. London: The Stationery Office; 2003.

26 Wells J and Bowers L. How prevalent is violence towards nurses working in general hospitals in the UK? *Journal of Advanced Nursing*. 2002; **39**: 230–40.

27 Department of Health. *We don't Have to Take This: NHS guidance on zero tolerance*. London: Department of Health; 1999.

28 Department of Health. 2000/2001 *Survey of Reported Violent or Abusive Incidents, Accidents Involving Staff and Sickness Absence in NHS Authorities, in England*. London: Department of Health; 2001.

29 Comptroller and Auditor General. *A Safer Place to Work: protecting NHS hospital and ambulance staff from violence and aggression.* London: The Stationery Office; 2003.

30 Commission for Health Improvement. *Commission for Health Improvement NHS Staff Survey.* London: Commission for Health Improvement; 2004.

31 Home Office. Criminal Statistics in England and Wales. London: HMSO; 2000.

32 Hoel H, Sparks K and Cooper C. *The Cost of Violence/Stress at Work and the Benefits of a Violence/Stress-free Working Environment.* Report commissioned by the International Labour Organisation, Geneva. Manchester: Institute of Science and Technology, University of Manchester; 2001.

33 National Institute of Occupational Safety and Health. NIOSH Current Intelligence Bulletin 57. *Violence in the Workplace: risk factors and prevention strategies.* London: National Institute of Occupational Safety and Health; 1996.

34 Atawneh FA, Zahid MA, Al-Sahlawi KS *et al.* Violence against nurses in hospitals: prevalence and effects. *British Journal of Nursing.* 2003; **12**: 102–107.

35 Whittington R, Shuttleworth S and Hill L. Violence to staff in a general hospital setting. *Journal of Advanced Nursing.* 1996; **24**: 326–33.

36 Ferns T and Chojnacka I. Reporting incidents of violence and aggression towards NHS staff. *Nursing Standard.* 2005; **19**: 51–6.

37 Shepherd J (ed). *Violence and Health Care Professionals.* London: Chapman and Hall; 1994.

38 Farrell GA. Therapeutic response to verbal abuse. *Nursing Standard.* 1992; **6**: 29–31.

39 Rew M and Ferns T. A balanced approach to dealing with violence and aggression at work. *British Journal of Nursing.* 2005; **14**: 227–32.

40 Shepherd J (ed). *Violence in Health Care: a practical guide to coping with violence and caring for victims.* Oxford: Oxford University Press; 1994.

41 Wykes T (ed). *Violence and Health Care Professionals.* London: Chapman and Hall; 1994.

42 Health Service Advisory Committee. *Violence and Aggression to Staff in Health Services.* Guidance on assessment and management. London: HSE Books; 1997.

43 Baron RA and Neuman J. Workplace violence and workplace aggression: evidence on their frequency and potential causes. *Aggressive Behaviour.* 1996; **22**: 161–73.

44 Mayhew C. Occupational violence in industrialised countries: types, incidence patterns, and 'at risk' groups of workers. In: Gill M, Fisher B and Bowie V (eds). *Occupational Violence in Industrialised Countries.* London: Willan Press; 2002.

45 Bulatao EQ and VandenBos GR. Workplace violence: its scope and the issues. In: VandenBos GR and Bulatao EQ (eds). *Violence on the Job.* Washington, DC: American Psychological Association; 1996.

46 Geddes D and Baron RA. Workplace aggression as a consequence of negative performance feedback. *Management Communication Quarterly.* 1997; **10**: 433–55.

47 Health and Safety Executive. *Reducing Risks – Protecting People.* London: HSE; 2004.

48 Eysneck HJ and Gudjonsson GH. *The Causes and Cures of Criminality.* New York: Plenum; 1989.

49 Rowett C. Violence in Social Work. Institute of Criminology, Occasional Paper No. 14, Cambridge: Cambridge University; 1986.

Chapter 2

Theories of aggression

Many theories of aggression have been developed, suggesting that there are many different causes of aggression. Each has its support and its criticism but although there is no unanimously accepted explanation, each theory helps to develop insight into the build-up and display of aggression. One division that does emerge is the question of whether violent behaviour results from factors that are beyond the perpetrator's control, or whether they are acts of free will and, therefore, largely preventable. The state of a perpetrator's physical or mental health may, for example, more readily explain acts of hitting, kicking or spitting that in other circumstances would be intolerable. Attempts at describing aggression are both diverse and often influenced by the professional discipline of the protagonist offering the explanation.[1] There would also seem to be a lack of meaning in much of the related terminology, and it appears that many of the views held result more from advocacy than evidence.

Biological theories of aggression

Biological theories of aggression have proved popular in trying to explain why some people become aggressive. Over the last decade, neuroscientists have made strides toward understanding the biology of violent behaviour. Research on both humans and animals has pointed to the important role of certain brain chemicals, especially the neurotransmitters serotonin and noradrenaline, in regulating aggressive impulses. Studies have shown that very low levels of serotonin are related to impulsive behaviour and explosive rages. Noradrenaline, in contrast, acts like an accelerator. High levels of this chemical within the brain are related to hyperarousal, in which a person might quickly over-react to even the slightest apparent threat. Unfortunately, though, a simple cause and effect relationship between these neurotransmitters has not in fact been found. So while they do not cause aggression on their own, they may contribute to the severity of the aggressive episode.[2,3]

In addition to the above, certain areas of the brain, the limbic system and cerebral cortex in particular, have been found to be responsible for aggressive emotions. Harper-Jaques and Reimer propose the term 'emotional circuit' to describe the interrelationship between the emotional processes of the limbic system and the neurocognitive processes of the frontal lobe and other parts of the cerebral cortex.[4] The functioning of this system is hypothesised to determine the meaning a person gives to a particular situation. Thus meaning is influenced by physiological capability to perceive incoming messages, to prioritise among competing stimuli, to interpret them in relation to stored ideas, beliefs and memories, and subsequently to respond. Abnormalities, congenital defects, tumours etc, in these areas of the brain have been linked to aggressive behaviour within the sufferer.

The endocrine system

Most research into hormones and the aggressive response has concerned the sex hormones. These are thought to act at two levels:

- first, by predisposing the individual to become biologically developed in terms of muscular and other body systems, to enable aggression to be used in the pursuit of sexual or other drives
- second, by the direct incitement to act aggressively under the influence of sexual hormones.

Owens and Ashcroft noted how the male sex hormone, androgen, influenced aggressive responses.[3] They discussed how castrated rats became less aggressive – probably due to their removed androgen supply – and how monkeys with high serum androgen concentrations were associated with higher levels of aggressive responses. The problem is that it is difficult to replicate these findings in human subjects. Although it can be shown that male delinquency is associated with the onset of puberty, attributing such behaviour to high androgen levels has not been proven in human subjects.[2]

One other area of hormonal influence on aggressive behaviour is the role of hormones in the menstrual cycle.[5] This was promoted by women attributing violent or aggressive actions to the premenstrual stage of their menstrual cycle (also *see* Chapter 7). Again a problem establishing a definite causal linkage is a major issue, and as yet this has not been established.

Genetic factors

Owens and Ashcroft identified three major genetic influences on aggressive behaviour:

- certain abnormal chromosome patterns influence aggressive behaviour
- personality has been considered to be genetically determined
- specific sex chromosomal abnormalities are associated with aggression, with some patterns increasing and others decreasing aggressive behaviour.[3]

Eysenck and Gudjonsson argued for a genetic influence in offending, as monozygotic (identical) twins were found to be more likely to offend than dizygotic (fraternal) twins.[6] Although this may be explained by similarities of upbringing rather than genetic factors, Bouchard *et al.* found that twins raised apart demonstrated similar behaviour.[7]

Jeffery also attributed aggressive behaviour to genetic make-up.[8] He considered that an extra Y chromosome in male prisoners was associated with aggressive behaviour. Additionally, he considered there were also a greater proportion of such individuals in secure hospital. The findings of this research have been questioned, however, as other studies have found that such individuals commit crime against property rather than against people.[9,10] Consequently, a similar problem emerges to that of other biological explanations of aggression. It is difficult to separate factors like genetic make-up from the complex variables that make up human individuals. Siann argued that to adhere strictly to a biological causation of aggression is inadequate because biological control of aggression is complex and incompletely understood.[11]

Ethological theories of aggression

Biological theories of aggression have also been advanced by ethologists, researchers who study the behaviour of animals in their natural environments. In doing so, several have advanced views about aggression in humans based on animal behaviour. This is done with the assumption that observations derived from the study of organisms below humans in the evolutionary scale will provide insight into human behaviour as well.

When ethologists consider any class of behaviour, they are, according to Hinde (1998), concerned with four issues, which are:

- what immediately causes it – this includes specific stimuli called releasers which trigger instinctive patterns of behaviour, and some of these are known as 'fixed action patterns'
- how such behaviour has developed over the animal's lifecycle (ontogeny)
- what the useful consequences of such behaviour are (its function)
- how the behaviour has evolved within the species (phylogeny).[12]

This view of aggression as an innate instinct in both humans and animals was popularised in three widely read books of the 1960s: *On Aggression* by Konrad Lorenz, *The Territorial Imperative* by Robert Ardrey and *The Naked Ape* by Desmond Morris.[13–15] The aggressive instinct postulated by these authors builds up spontaneously – with or without provocation – until it is likely to be discharged with minimal or no provocation from outside stimuli. In addition, Lorenz suggested that man's social evolution means that aggressive tendencies and feelings of aggression build up inside us and are not released through everyday activities as they were in our evolutionary past in activities such as hunting.[13] He argued that we expend very little energy just staying alive and get a build-up of aggression by thinking about life's problems and stressors. He also went on to argue that aggression also has an adaptive function, allowing us to deal with changes to our living environment and to 'evolve'. What Lorenz and others failed to account for was the variation in aggressiveness from person to person and culture to culture.

Psychosocial theories of aggression

Three major psychological theories of aggression are considered here:

- psychoanalytic theory
- frustration–aggression hypothesis
- social learning theory.

The psychoanalytic theory of aggression

Psychoanalytic theorists view emotions as instinctual urges. Suppressing these urges is viewed as unhealthy and may contribute to the development of psycho-somatic or psychological disorders. Freud struggled to understand the nature and expression of human aggressive behaviour. In his early works, he linked aggression with libidinal factors. He considered aggression to be instinctual and inevitable. According to Freud, the aim of all instincts is to reduce tension or excitation to a minimum and eventually to its total elimination, thus allowing humans to return to the idyllic state previously enjoyed within the womb.[16] The only way of achieving this is through a state of nothingness from which it had emerged, in other words death.[17,18] However, this association did not explain destructive actions that occurred during the wars and armed conflict. In his latter writings, Freud identified aggression as a separate instinct, like the sexual instinct. In doing so, he challenged the commonly held belief that human beings were essentially good. Instead, he viewed aggression as an innate human quality that could be expressed when a person was provoked or abused.[19] Freud's view fostered the use of catharsis, the release of ideas through talking and expressing appropriate emotion.

Erich Fromm (1900–1980) an American psychoanalyst best known for his application of psychoanalytic theory to social and cultural problems, held a different view. He believed that animals and humans shared one form of aggression that he called benign. This was a genetically programmed response designed as a defence mechanism to protect the person against threat. However, unlike animals, human beings were capable of behaving aggressively for other reasons. He defined aggression in humans as any behaviour that causes or intends to cause damage to another person, to an animal, or to an object.[20] The distinction made between humans and animals was that the human could reason. This capability provides them with options that are not available to animals. Humans may foresee both real and perceived threats. Perceived threats that are based on distorted perceptions may lead to aggressive and violent behaviours.

Frustration–aggression hypothesis

The frustration–aggression hypothesis was first set out in the 1930s by Dollard *et al.* in an attempt to translate some of Freud's psychoanalytic concepts into learning theory.[21] It was proposed that aggression, rather than occurring spontaneously for no reason, is the response to the frustration of some goal-directed behaviour by an outside source. Goals may include such basic needs as food, water, sleep, sex, love and recognition.

Aggression from this source does have limitations however, including inhibition, fear of retaliation etc. Likewise, people may respond in other ways, sometimes becoming passive and helpless in extreme cases. One form of this view is the concept of displacement of aggression, where a substitute object is found for the expression of aggressive feelings because they cannot be vented openly and directly towards their real target.[16] For example, an employee who is rebuked by his or her superior may in turn displace their feelings of anger onto a junior member of staff. In this sense the urge to behave aggressively is not lost but displaced until a more suitable time and target is available.

This bears some similarity to the concept of *scapegoating*, since a scapegoat is:

1 relatively powerless to retaliate to acts of aggression
2 made to take the blame for actions which he, she or the group is not responsible.[22]

Contributions to frustration–aggression research further established that an environmental stimulus must produce not just frustration but anger in order for aggression to follow, and that the anger can be the result of stimuli other than frustrating situations, such as verbal abuse. That is not to say that anger will always lead to aggression, however, as anger can be displayed in a number of ways and, conversely, act as a motivator and medium for positive change.

This model of aggression has been heavily criticised, however, on the grounds of providing an over-simplistic account of aggression. In addition, the concept of frustration is loosely specified and does not adequately predict which types of frustrating experience lead to aggression.

Social learning theory

In contrast to instinct theories, social learning theory focuses on aggression as a learnt behaviour. This approach stresses the roles that social influences, such as models and reinforcement, play in the acquisition of aggressive behaviour.

Social learning has three principal components:

1 *behaviour*: an observer sees a model perform a particular behaviour
2 *learning or acquisition phase*: the observer attends to important features of the behaviour, remembering what was seen and done
3 *performance*: imitates the behaviour at a later time.

Bandura suggested that much aggressive behaviour is learnt by observing and imitating others and by being rewarded and punished.[23] Aggressive children often have parents who model aggressive behaviour. Parents who have been abused themselves often pass on this behaviour to their own children, through observational learning, imitation etc. People can learn the rewards of aggression, for instance a child whose aggressive behaviour successfully intimidates other children will more than likely become increasingly aggressive.[24]

Children have also been found to pick up aggressive styles of acting in films etc very quickly, but they do not usually portray this immediately, unless it will give them an obvious advantage.[25] The information seems to be stored because it may be useful later on, and it is this, 'delay', that has caused much concern for censors. Any behaviour that is rewarded or reinforced is more likely to occur in the future.

The social learning view of aggression is that the emotional arousal stemming from an aversive experience motivates aggression. Whether aggression or some other response actually occurs depends on what consequences we have learned to expect. Theories of aggression based on instinct and frustration assume that hostile urges erupt from inner emotions, which naturally push aggression from within us. Social psychologists contend that learning also 'pulls' aggression out of us. Reducing restraints on aggressive behaviour through modelling can reduce the inhibitions against behaving aggressively, by coming to believe that this is a typical or permissible way of solving problems or attaining goals, and, in turn, this distort a person's views about conflict resolution.[26–28]

Cognitive theory

Cognitive theorists are interested in how people transform internal and external stimuli into useful information. Emphasis is placed on understanding how the person takes new information and fits it into an already developed schema. Beck proposed that an angry response is influenced by cognitive schema such as judgements, self-esteem and expectations (*see* Figure 2.1 below).[29] In a situation perceived as intentional, dangerous or unprovoked, the recipient's reaction will be intensified. The person's reaction will be further intensified if the offender is viewed as undesirable. In psychological disorders, cognitive processing may be compromised. Anger is regarded as an inappropriate negative emotion because it stems from irrational beliefs. Change is directed at altering irrational beliefs by identifying them and working to change them and the associated psychological processes.

The relationship between thoughts, feelings and behaviour is shown in Figure 2.1.

Hostile and instrumental aggression

Attempts to classify aggression into various categories have not necessarily clarified this hugely disparate and complex collection of philosophical, biological, sociological and psychological interpretations of our behaviour.

Moyer and Moyer presented an early, and highly influential, classification of eight different forms of aggression based upon the stimulus precipitating them. These are:[31]

- *predatory aggression*: this aggression is directed to natural prey and is deeply rooted in our ancestors' hunting behaviour. Today it can be seen in the behaviour of those who view a particular person or group as less important than them

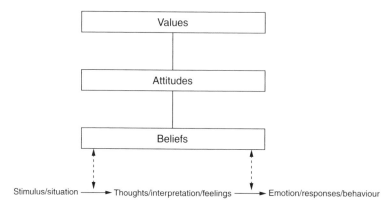

Figure 2.1 The relationship between thoughts, feelings and beliefs.[30]

- *inter-male aggression*: the physical violence or submissive behaviour displayed by males towards each other. Possible causes for such violence could be perceived competition for resources and ego threats that one male feels are being created by a second male
- *fear-induced aggression*: responses believed to be biologically programmed into us so that we act in an aggressive manner towards any form of forced confinement
- *territorial aggression*: threat or attack behaviour displayed towards an invasion of territory or the submissive-retreat behaviour displayed when confronted while intruding on another's territory. Invasion of territory can include much more than property but also power and status
- *maternal aggression*: aggressive behaviour put forward by females (and most likely males as well) when an intruder is in the presence of offspring
- *irritable aggression*: aggression and rage directed towards an object when the aggressor is frustrated, hurt, deprived, or stressed
- *sex-related aggression*: aggressive behaviour that is elicited by the same stimuli that elicit sexual behaviour. Any person who can evoke sexual desire can equally evoke aggression via jealousy, etc. Besides the obvious jealousy–violence reactions, some individuals may for one reason or another come to associate sexual desire with violence and dominance. This association could possibly explain a number of violent sexual acts that occur
- *instrumental aggression*: aggressive behaviour displayed because it previously resulted in a reward. Much of human aggression seems to be related to this. If a person has received a reward (money, sexual gratification) due to a deviant aggressive act that they had performed, they will be conditioned towards committing that act again when they are motivated to obtain that previously possessed reward.

It seems clear that many of these categories overlap; for example, fear-induced aggression may be caused by an aggressor attempting to harm the young of the victim, thus causing fear and aggression (maternal, territorial and fear-induced aggression).

Ramirez used three categories:[32]

- *inter-specific aggression*: equivalent to Moyer's predatory aggression
- *intra-specific aggression*: including most of the aggression seen in social inter-actions and which comprises inter-male, territorial, maternal aggression and sex-related aggression
- *indiscriminate or reactive aggression*: which is largely defensive in character and consists of categories such as fear-induced aggression.

The role of anger

While anger frequently precedes violent behaviour, it is important to recognise that anger does not always lead to violence.[33] Friedman and Booth-Kewley defined anger as an immediate emotional arousal to a given or perceived situation, hostility as a more enduring negative attitude and aggression as the actual or intended harming of others.[34] It is one of the negative emotions that occurs when there is a threat, delay, or thwarting of a goal, or a conflict between goals.[35]

Anger offers a signal to those experiencing the emotion that something is wrong in themselves, in others, or in their relationship(s) with others.[36] Thomas suggests that the experience of anger can be used as a warning signal that demands greater than available resources.[37] With the exception of anger that arises from specific neurological damage or biochemical imbalances, angry episodes can be viewed as social events.[38] The meaning of angry episodes develops from the beliefs held about anger and the interpretation given to the episode.[39] The three possible targets of a person's anger are others, impersonal objects/life conditions, or oneself.[39]

Sometimes it may be therapeutic to legitimise anger, perhaps if the standard of healthcare falls below what the individual expects. In fact, many people believe that anger is healthy and necessary. Towl and Crighton suggest that it is a common experience to become angry, and that expressing anger is a normal process.[40] It is not the anger that is legitimate and right, but the stress that underlies the anger.[41] Expressing anger is also a mechanism for enhancing self-respect, and a constructive action that can lead to correcting a perceived wrong.[42]

Anger is believed to play several roles in aggression:[43-45]

- anger reduces inhibitions and increases the chance of the person using aggression as a means of expression
- in turn, anger can sometimes provide a justification for aggressive retaliation by interfering with moral reasoning and judgement
- anger allows a person to maintain an aggressive intention over time. It increases attention to the provoking events, increases the depth of processing of those events, and therefore improves recall of those events. In this way, anger allows a person to reinstate the state that was present in the originally provoking situation
- anger (like other emotions) is used as an information cue. It informs people about causes, culpability, and possible ways of responding (e.g. retaliation). If anger is triggered in an ambiguous social situation, the anger experience itself helps resolve the ambiguities, and does so in the direction of hostile interpretations
- anger primes aggressive thoughts, scripts, and associated expressive-motor behaviours. Such anger-related knowledge structures are used to interpret the situation and to provide aggressive responses to the situation. One related consequence of the many links between anger and various knowledge structures is that people frequently pay more attention to anger-related stimuli than to similar neutral stimuli
- lastly, anger energises behaviour by increasing arousal levels.

Activity 2.1

What makes you angry? List the things that make you feel hostile or aggressive. Make a list of how you might go about reducing these feelings and how you could respond to them differently, if at all.

There are several other features of human aggression that must be successfully explained by any 'general' model. For instance, one powerful predictor of aggression is opportunity, or the social situation. Some situations restrict opportunities to aggress; others provide opportunities. Most people do not commit extreme acts of violence even if they could do so with little chance of discovery or punishment.[46] Such self-regulation is due, in large part, to the fact that people cannot easily escape the moral standards that they apply to themselves. Self-image, self-standards, and a sense of self-worth are used in normal self-regulation behaviour. However, people with apparently normal moral standards sometimes behave reprehensibly towards others by committing such acts as murder, torture and cruelty.[47]

References

1 Baron RA. Social and personal determinants of workplace aggression: evidence for the impact of percived injustice and the Type A behavior pattern. *Aggressive Behaviour*. 1999; **25**: 281–96.

2 Hollin CR. *Criminal Behaviour*. London: The Farmer Press; 1992.

3 Owens RG and Ashcroft JB. *Violence: a guide for the caring professions*. London: Croom; 1995.

4 Harper-Jaques S and Reimer M. Biopsychosocial management of aggression and violence. In: Boyd MA and Nihart MA (eds). *Psychiatric Nursing*. New York: Lippincott-Raven; 1998.

5 Prentky R. The neurochemistry and neuroendocrinology of sexual aggression. In: Farrington DP and Gunn J (eds). *Aggression and Dangerousness*. London: John Wiley; 1985.

6 Eysneck HJ and Gudjonsson GH. *The Causes and Cures of Criminality*. New York: Plenum; 1989.

7 Bouchard TJ, Lykken DT, McGue M *et al*. Sources of human psychological differences: the Minnesota study of twins reared apart. *Science*. 1990; **350**: 223–28.

8 Jeffery CR. *Biology and Crime*. London: Sage Publications; 1979.

9 Casey MD, Blank CE, McLean TM *et al*. Male patients with chromosome abnormality in the state hospitals. *Journal of Mental Deficiency Research*. 1973; **16**: 215–56.

10 Price WH. Sex chromosome abnormalities in special hospital patients. In: Owens RG and Ashcroft JB (eds). *Violence: a Guide for the Caring Professions*. London: Croom; 1995.

11 Siann G. Accounting for aggression: perspectives on aggression and violence. In: Brennan W. Aggression and violence: examining the theories. *Nursing Standard*. 1998; **12**: 36–8.

12 Hinde RA. Ethology. In: Brennan W. Aggression and violence: examining the theories. *Nursing Standard*. 1998; **12**: 36–8.

13 Lorenz K. *On Aggression*. London: Harcourt Brace Jovanovich; 1966.

14 Ardrey R. *The Territorial Imperative*. London: Fontanna; 1969.

15 Morris D. *The Naked Ape*. New York: McGraw-Hill; 1967.

16 Gross R. *Psychology: the science of mind and behaviour*. London: Hodder and Stoughton; 1992.

17 Buss A. *Personality: temperament, social behviour and the self*. Boston: Allyn and Bacon; 1998.

18 Frankl G. *The Unknown Self*. London: Open Gate Press; 1990.

19 Davidson RJ, Scherer K and Goldsmith HH (eds). *Handbook of Affective Sciences*. Oxford: Oxford University Press; 2001.

20 Fromm E. *The Anatomy of Human Destructiveness*. Harmondsworth: Penguin; 1973.

21 Dollard J, Doob L, Miller NE *et al. Frustration and Aggression*. New Haven: Yale University Press; 1939.

22 Ohon N. Workplace violence: theories of causation and prevention strategies. *Journal of the American Association of Occupational Health Nurses*. 1994; **4**: 477–82.

23 Bandura A. *Social Learning Theory*. New Jersey: Prentice Hall; 1977.

24 Bandura A. *Principles of Behaviour Modification*. New York: Holt; 1969.

25 Bandura A, Ross D and Ross SA. Imitation of film-meditated aggressive models. *Journal of of Abnormal and Social Psychology*. 1963; **42**: 63–6.

26 Bushman BJ. Moderating role of trait aggressiveness in the effects of violent media on aggression. *Journal of Personality and Social Psychology*. 1995; **69**: 950–60.

27 Bushman BJ. Priming effects of violent media on the accessibility of aggressive constructs in memory. *Personality and Social Psychology Bulletin*. 1998; **24**: 537–45.

28 Geen RG. *Human Aggression* (2e). New York: Taylor and Francis; 2001.

29 Mischel W and Shoda Y. A cognitive-affective system theory of personaility: reconceptulizing situations, dispositions, dynamics, and invariance in personality structure. *Psychological Review*. 1995; **102**: 246–68.

30 Nelson H. *Cognitive Behavioural Therapy with Schizophrenia: a practice manual*. London: Nelson Thornes; 1997.

31 Moyer K and Moyer KE. *The Psychology of Aggression*. New York: Harper and Row; 1976.

32 Ramirez JM. The nature of aggression in animals. In: Brennan W. Aggression and violence: examining the theories. *Nursing Standard*. 1998; **12**: 36–8.

33 Hollinworth H, Clark C, Harland R *et al*. Understanding the arousal of anger: a patient-centred approach. *Nursing Standard*. 2005; **19**: 41–7.

34 Friedman H and Booth-Kewley S. The 'disease-prone personality'. A meta-analytic view of the construct. *American Psychologist*. 1987; **42**: 539–55.

35 Higgins E and Kruglanski A (eds). *Social Psychology: handbook of basic principles*. New York: Guildford Press; 1996.

36 Lerner HG. *Women in Therapy*. New Jersey: Jason Aronson Publishers; 1988.

37 Thomas SP. *Transforming Nurses' Anger and Pain: steps towards healing*. New York: Springer; 1998.

38 Travis C. *Anger: the misuderstood emotion* (2e). New York: Touchstone; 1989.

39 Carlson M, Marcus-Newhall A and Miller N. Effects of situational aggression cues: a quantative review. *Journal of Personality and Social Psychology*. 1990; **58**: 622–33.

40 Towl GJ and Crighton DA. *The Handbook of Psychology for Forensic Practitioners*. New York: Routledge; 1996.

41 McKay M, Rogers P and McKay J. *When Anger Hurts: quieting the storm within*. Oakland: New Harbinger Publications; 1989.

42 Turkel A. The 'voice of self-respect': women and anger. *Journal of the American Academy of Psychoanalysis*. 2000; **28**: 527–40.

43 Geen RG and Donnerstein E (eds). *Human Aggression: theories, research and implications for policy*. New York: Academic Press; 1998.

44 Huesmann LR. An information-processing model for the development of aggression. *Aggressive Behavior*. 1988; **14**: 13–24.

45 Berkowitz L. On the formation and regulation of anger and aggression: a cognative-neoassociationistic analysis. *American Psychologist*. 1990; **45**: 494–503.

46 Simon LMJ. Does criminal offender treatment work? *Applied and Preventive Psychology*. 1998; **7**: 137–59.

47 Berkowitz L. Affect, aggression and antisocial behaviour. In: Davidson K, Scherer K and Goldsmith HH (eds). *Handbook of Affective Sciences*. Oxford: Oxford University Press; 2001.

Chapter 3

Managing violence and aggression: risk reduction and prevention

Responding to violence and aggression

The issue of responding to and managing violence and aggression is one of the major challenges facing modern health services.[1-3] There would appear to be no simple answer to the problem. During the course of the last 10–15 years there has been a variety of strategies and recommendations put forward for the healthcare industry by governmental agencies and violence experts, which have met with differing degrees of success. Research into the effectiveness of such actions is lacking, and there is confusion as to what constitutes best practice.[4] Some of the strategies used in managing violence and aggression would seem to contradict each other, and may in themselves prompt aggression if not used properly.

Safe systems of work

The recommended approach to managing violence and aggression in the workplace is to eliminate the opportunity of it occurring (risk prevention). If such behaviour cannot be prevented, planning should focus on reducing the impact on the people, the workplace and the work processes (risk reduction and risk management). Staff should be prepared and confident that they will know what to do if a violent incident occurs. A safe system of work is a formal procedure, which results from a systematic examination of the task in order to identify all the hazards and assess the risks. It also identifies safe methods of work, to ensure that the hazards are eliminated or the remaining risks are minimised.

Developing a safe system of work

A safe system of work encompasses the following:

- *hazard identification*: identify situations where staff and visitors may be injured or harmed
- *risk assessment*: identify the extent to which staff and visitors may be injured or harmed
- *risk control*: implement safe methods of work based on the findings of risk assessment
- *monitor and review of the system*: regularly check the implementation and effectiveness of the risk control measures.

Hazard identification

This part of the process is about identifying possible situations where staff and other people may be physically or psychologically harmed by violent or aggressive behaviour. This may not always be obvious as staff will often hide their concerns. In compiling a list of hazards it is important to include information from near-miss incidents where no one was actually hurt but the potential for harm was there. This can often be useful in preventing a future more serious occurrence. Since violence will vary according to area, it is essential that this exercise is carried out at a local level with the staff group concerned; for instance, staff working in mental health face different risks from those working in an area such as paediatrics where the relatives will usually pose a greater risk than the patient. Decide who might be harmed and how; remember to think about people who may not be in the workplace all the time, for example visitors and maintenance staff.

Risk assessment

Risk assessment involves gathering information from multiple sources and informants with the focus on identifying the factors associated with an increased probability of risk behaviour happening.[5] In addition to being good practice, the assessment and management of risk is a legal requirement, and failure to complete an adequate risk assessment could lead to enforcement action by the Health and Safety Executive (*see* Chapter 8). In assessing the level of risk, there is a need to take account of both the likelihood and the potential consequences of each violent incident. Enough information is needed to understand the factors which could escalate violent behaviour and make the situation worse.

The following questions may prove useful when thinking about risk:[6]

- how serious is the risk?
- is the risk specific or general?
- how immediate is the risk?
- how volatile is the risk?

Remember the potential effects on staff of repeated severe verbal abuse or threats. Continued exposure to verbal abuse can create high levels of stress and anxiety, reduce the morale of staff, and lead to sickness and absence.

Having undertaken a risk assessment it is important that this is recorded. This might include:

- the hazards identified – potential assailants and high-risk areas
- the staff groups exposed to risks
- the existing preventive measures
- an evaluation of the remaining risks
- any additional preventative or control measures identified.

Risk control

Having analysed the risks involved, there is a need to check whether the precautions already in place are adequate for the job. If they are not and significant risks remain, more will need to be done. Preventative measures should always be considered and developed first with the aim of eliminating the risk entirely. For example, if the risk arises from carrying drugs, make other arrangements for their delivery. However, there are no ready-made solutions to prevent violence, and any proposed action must be relevant to the particular workplace under consideration. In this way, the wearing of a uniform may be a risk factor for community staff working in some districts but not others.

Where hazards cannot be eliminated and risks reduced, a safe method of work should be devised. When a system has been developed, it then has to be implemented – this can be done verbally or by written instructions – for example, work policies and procedures. There must be adequate communication if the safe system of work is to be successful. The details should be understood by everyone who has to work with it, and must be carried out on each occasion. It is important that everyone appreciates the need for the system and its place in the accident prevention programme. Where training and instruction are required then these should be provided and include all the necessary skills, awareness of the system, and the hazards the programme is aiming to eliminate by the use of the safe procedures.

Monitoring the system

Effective monitoring requires that regular checks are made to ensure that the system is still appropriate for the needs of the task, and that it is still being complied with. Active monitoring involves checking that systems and procedures are working, without waiting until something goes wrong. Reactive monitoring involves looking at incidents after the event and helps everyone learn from the experience. This depends on an effective system of reporting and recording incidents. The minority of trusts that use a specific aggression and violence reporting form enjoy a greater use of information feedback into the management and training structure to effect change and improvements in staff safety.

Systems such as preventative measures will need to be analysed for their success, for example whether they have prevented or controlled the risk, or whether they have had any adverse effect. Training should be monitored and reviewed to see whether it is appropriate and effective. Successful actions can help to persuade staff that the policy is effective.

If monitoring has shown that a measure has no obvious benefit, then there is a need to reassess the problem and try other measures. There are likely to be occasions when a number of measures may need to be tested before a final solution is found. If a measure is unsuccessful, it may be necessary to remove it completely. Sometimes a simple modification may be all that is required to enable it to be effective.

Audit

Audit provides an independent assessment of the systems in place. Employers may choose to carry out an internal audit or engage independent auditors to provide a check on the reliability, efficiency, and effectiveness of the performance measures contained within the operating system. Audit is an important part in the role of managing violence and aggression:[7]

- it informs the guidance development process, providing information on the current position in relation to evidence-based standards
- it provides information on the benefits associated with implementation and the resulting improvements in patient care
- after initial audits, re-audits can highlight the changes in practice and their effectiveness
- it ensures a level of quality within the system.

Consulting staff

Consulting and involving staff in all the activities above can have significant benefit:[8]

- it will show a genuine commitment to tackling the problem
- it will ensure that any reporting or monitoring scheme is practical and effective
- the knowledge and experience of staff are valuable resources when deciding on practical preventative and protective measures
- staff who have been fully consulted will have a stronger commitment in helping to implement the policy and measures.

Focus on individual risk assessment

The purpose of any risk assessment is to provide information on which to make decisions that allow risk factors to be minimised and appropriately managed.[9] Risk needs to be differentiated from dangerousness, with risk being the likelihood of an event occurring and dangerousness being the degree of harm that may occur should the event happen.[10] This is an important point, as the risk may be infrequent but the consequences of it happening may be such that it requires constant monitoring and intervention.

Risk assessment for violence and aggression can be regarded as a function of four factors:[11]

- the frequency of potential conflict situations
- the duration of the conflict situation
- the likelihood of the individuals involved acting in a violent or aggressive manner
- the magnitude of the harm caused.

Key risk areas include:[12]

- harm to others
- harm to self
- neglect of self
- exploitation of others

One person alone cannot do an adequate risk assessment, and information should be gathered from a number of sources and shared. In addition to this, it is important to recognise that risk is dynamic in nature and is largely dependent on circumstance, which can alter over a brief period of time. Because of this risk, assessment needs to be predominately short-term, and subject to frequent review and, as such, time should be made for gathering, discussing and analysing information.

Individual risk assessment

Great emphasis is placed on getting to know the patient. A good relationship with the patient allows the healthcare worker to understand the patient and to detect changes in their behaviour, which may be suggestive of possible aggression or violence, and guide actions with specific individuals. An assessment of individual risk should include the following:[9]

- history of behaviour(s)
- recency
- severity
- frequency
- pattern
- ideation/thought content
- affect/mood
- planned intent.

The reason to examine past history is to establish facts, clarify patterns of behaviour and make clear their context. Past behaviour is the best indicator of future behaviour, and time should be spent exploring this.

Useful questions in assessing individual risk include:[13]

- how likely is it that a patient will act in a violent way?
- in what way?
- in what circumstances?
- to what is the likelihood related?
- what is the severity of the risk?
- what is the frequency of the risk?
- how long is the risk of violence likely to last?

Sources of information include:

- access to past records
- self-reports at interview
- observing discrepancies between verbal and non-verbal cues (*see* Chapter 4)
- reports from significant others/formal and informal discussions
- rating scales/descriptive reports
- intuitive gut reactions (vital clues, but not easily documented)
- recognising repeating patterns of behaviour.

Common errors in failing to identify risk include:[14]

- minimisation of historical events in the patient's case file
- over-reliance on recent progress

- sudden changes of view in the care team
- extraneous factors not openly recognised (resources, fear, unpopularity, singularly strong opinions)
- infrequency/discontinuity of assessment
- non-verification of statements made by patients or others
- not taking account of evidence contrary to the patient's assertions
- not recognising patient manipulation and consequent staff discord
- lack of thorough investigation and assessment of assertions of insight and remorse
- discounting information if not supportive of hoped for outcomes
- avoiding confrontation with the client.

Table 3.1 gives examples of factors in the individual that are predictive of aggression.[15-17] However, individual factors are not enough when predicting the likelihood of risk. Consideration also needs to be given to the nature and motive of the interaction between members of staff and the patient, and the environment and context in which the intervention takes place. Risk factors then may be viewed from the standpoint of:

- the environment
- administration and work practices
- the patient and healthcare worker.

Table 3.1 Prediction of aggression: the individual (adapted from Farrington, 1994; Hinde, 1993 and Pollock *et al.*, 1989[15-17]

Prediction category	Examples
Personality factors	Low threshold of frustration or impulsivity Increased liability to become aroused An antisocial personality such as someone who is habitually aggressive or under-controlled Substance abusers
Previous history of aggression or violence	An institutional record where violence has been a factor may mean an increased risk of violence A genetic constitution that tends towards a lack of control
Biological factors	Disinhibitory factors such as caused by brain damage, and some organic mental illnesses
Mental disorder	Psychotic individuals who experience a build-up of tension before a violent outburst Some depressed individuals may attempt to kill others for altruistic reasons, to relieve their supposed suffering Frustration, fear or pain may lead to aggressive responses

Table 3.2 Prediction of aggression: the social environment (adapted from Farrington, 1994; Hinde, 1993 and Pollock *et al.*, 1989[15-17]

Prediction category	Examples
Peer influences and group pressures	Peer and group pressures to act aggressively may be exerted on individuals Certain geographical areas may process more aggressive cues than others
Economic, social and environmental influences	Economic and social deprivation tend to be associated with offending and sometimes aggressive responses There may be an association between situational influences and aggressive behaviour, such as the availability of weapons Additional social factors include extra-familial roles, peer group and media influences Uncomfortable or stressful social or physical conditions can predispose an individual to aggression
The presence of a target	The assertion is made here that aggression is not likely to occur without the presence of a target

If the reason for potential violence and aggression can be identified, and if it can be changed, there is a greater chance that the amount of this type of behaviour can be reduced. Having identified a risk, the healthcare worker has a responsibility to take action with a view to ensuring that the risk is reduced and managed effectively; this might be a simple measure of reporting it and ensuring that action is taken. Table 3.2 gives examples of factors in the social environment that are predictive of aggression.[15-17]

Risk management

Risk management is the process of planning and decision making, including the identification and development of strategies that reduce the severity and frequency of identified adverse risks.[18] Actions to reduce the identified risk can then be taken, based on the findings of the risk assessment. These actions may include relatively small measures such as removing from a room ornaments that could be used as weapons, to more major measures such as providing closed circuit television units (CCTV) and the monitoring of clinical areas. It is important to remember that what works to reduce or prevent one type of violence may have limited use upon another type. The management plan should change the balance between risk and safety, following the principle of negotiating safety.

Individual risk management plans

An individual risk management plan provides a link between risk assessment information and the known or potential interventions. It contains clear statements of anticipated risk and how it can be avoided or its impact minimised. In order for staff members to identify and deal effectively with patients who behave in a violent and aggressive manner, individual risk management plans should be in place that include a gradual progression on measures to prevent violent behaviour from escalating. Such risk management plans should be made with input from all levels of care providers as appropriate. Effective plans and procedures would cover verbal or physical threats. Such plans call for creative thinking, in order to promote what is termed positive risk taking, supporting individual choice and decision making and helping the patient regain control of their situation. Again such plans of care should be articulated in policy and procedure as they relate to the circumstances of the service user.

A risk management plan should:

- provide a link between risk assessment information and the known or potential interventions
- contain clear statements of anticipated risk and how it can be avoided or its impact minimised
- demonstrate detailed knowledge of a person's history and early warning signs of risk, with responses to potential or anticipated risk
- give an articulation of policies and procedures as they relate to the circumstances of a service user
- provide a guide for monitoring progress
- detail crisis responses to real situations of clinical risk
- demonstrate creative thinking to promote positive risk taking (supporting individual choice and decision making) in an area of practice dominated by negative and restrictive responses.

Box 3.1   Risk management: representation

Personal signs and situational context = increased probability of ...... for which ...... are possible interventions.

For example:

If X is in ...... situation /with ......, then he/she is likely to behave in the following ways: ......

The early signs of these processes are commonly ...... (thoughts/ behaviours) and the risk of ...... is then significantly increased.

In these circumstances, the following interventions ...... have proved most effective (with ...... being the least effective).

Prevention

Prevention is essentially about using all available information to ensure that the risk of future incidents can be minimised. This includes learning from operational experience of previous incidents and adopting an inclusive approach that involves staff and stakeholders. It is therefore, essential that staff are encouraged to report identified risks to managers, as well as incidents that have or may have occurred, so that appropriate action can be taken.

Prevention of harm takes place at two levels.[19] At the first level, the aim is basically to prevent acts of violence from occurring, or at least to reduce them (*see* Table 3.3). At the second level, if the act of violence has occurred, support is required for the person who has experienced the incident. This support should seek to minimise the harmful effects of the incident on both a practical and emotional level.

Table 3.3   The prevention of harm

Preventive actions	*Examples*
Workplace environment	• Consideration of physical security measures, for example, entry locks, screens, adequate lighting, reception desks, emergency exits, installation of video surveillance systems, alarm systems, coded doors, elimination or limitation of no-exit areas, and objects which could serve as projectiles • Provision of better setting, décor, regular information about delays etc
Work organisation and job design	• Improved reception and public information • Sufficient staff • Check visitors' credentials • Avoiding lone work and where this is not possible, keeping in touch with lone workers
Staff training and information	• To recognise unacceptable behaviour and the early warning signs of aggression • How to manage difficult situations • To follow procedures set up to protect employees such as to apply security instructions, to ensure adequate communication, to act to reduce a person's aggression, to identify clients with a history of violence • To manage the stress inherent in the situation in order to control emotional reactions

It is likely that you will need a mixture of preventative measures to achieve control and manage the problem effectively. It is important that they are appropriate and adequate for the task and cost-effective. However, prevention is a complex process, and approaches that may be successful in reducing particular forms of aggression and violence may be counter-productive in dealing with different persons in different situations.

In developing precautions, you may find it helpful to ask yourself:[20]

- is there any way to change:
  - the jobs people do?
  - the circumstances in which they work?
  - the way jobs are done (for example, matching the length of appointments to the likely time of the consultation where possible can reduce waiting times, and in turn, stress and anxiety)?
  - the workplace?
  - the information given to employees and the way it is communicated?
  - the system for sharing information about patients?
  - the response to incidents?
  - the incident-recording system?
- is training directed at the risk and the relevant employees?
- are there support systems for employees that are confidential and accessible? Do they lead to a return to work?

Activity 3.1

- Reflect on the extent to which your employing authority protects you from potentially violent situations.
- Assess how this could be improved.
- Discuss with other members of staff strategies for preventing aggressive/ violent situations from developing. If you are able to anticipate aggression you are more likely to be able to prevent it. Remember that even the most skilled individual may become a target of violence, and while the organisation plays a significant role in preventing aggression and violence there is a need to develop personal strategies and skills to diffuse potential aggressive and violent situations.

Reporting

Documentation of violent incidents in the workplace is another form of preventative action. Collecting and analysing data (including near-misses) will help establish whether there is a pattern of incidents, and identify particular targets or practices at risk. However, each system needs to be tailored to fit the organisational structure and the type of work undertaken.

Burton stresses that the need for prompt and accurate recording of an aggressive incident is essential and should include every relevant detail, even before the incident occurred.[21] This will allow for investigation into the incident, but more importantly for remedial action to start quickly. The main aim of any system is to prevent similar incidents from occurring in the future, for example by identifying the need for changes to the workplace, changes to working procedures, or additional training requirements. The reporting of incidents also helps to identify trends, assist the review process, and inform risk assessments. Forms to gather such information need to be relevant to the particular employer's circumstances. It may be useful to collate information such as:[20]

- the number of incidents
- when they occur
- the types of staff involved
- the categories of patients involved
- the environments or locations where incidents happen
- the level of injuries sustained
- the preventative measures recommended.

A number of report forms already exist with some carrying a legal requirement for completion. The Reporting of Injuries, Diseases and Dangerous Occurrences Regulations, 1995 (RIDDOR) for example requires employers to notify their enforcing authority in the event of an accident at work to an employee. This includes any act of non-consensual physical violence done to a person at work. In addition to this, employers must also report cases in which employees have been off work for three working days or more following an assault that resulted in physical injury. Likewise, the Counter Fraud and Security Management Service (CFSMS) has also instigated a reporting system which managers are required to abide by in the event of a physical assault (*see* Box 3.2).[22]

Box 3.2 Counter Fraud and Security Management Directions for Reporting Incidents of Physical Aggression

Each NHS body must:

- nominate one of its executive directors to take responsibility for security management matters, including its particular responsibility for measures to deal with violence towards staff
- monitor and ensure compliance with CFSMS directives and inform all NHS staff of the content of these directives and what is required of them to ensure compliance
- take into account any other guidance or advice on measures to deal with violence against NHS staff which may be issued by the CSFMS.

In cases of physical assault the nominated director must ensure that:

- he or she is informed of the incident
- the police are contacted immediately either by the person assaulted or by an appropriate manager or colleague, and that full co-operation is given to the police in any investigation
- the CFSMS is informed of the incident and that full co-operation is given to it in any investigation or subsequent action which it considers appropriate
- the details are recorded in accordance with the NHS body's incident reporting system
- the victim of the assault is informed of the investigation's progress and offered such support as is necessary or desirable in the circumstances.

Environmental factors

The physical environment may affect the likelihood of violent and aggressive incidents and the ease with which people can respond to them.[23] Some areas of healthcare buildings need to be open to the public, but uncontrolled access to all areas may expose some staff to unnecessary risk. The overall design of a building should facilitate the treatment of patients and accommodate concerned relatives and friends.[24] However, violence can arise out of frustration or annoyance amongst other things, caused by a failure or general inadequacy of a building's design and its facilities. A poor physical environment suggests that neither patients nor staff are valued or cared for. The aim should be to make all work areas secure, well-lit, and protected from the likelihood of assaults.

Access to buildings should be controlled and monitored and, where possible, have a single point of entry/exit.[18] Patients and their relatives should not be left to wander aimlessly; a clear indication as to where they should proceed in order to seek help and assistance should be evident.

Areas should be kept clean and hospitable, and above all welcoming, particularly reception and waiting rooms. Thought should go into the decoration of units, colour scheme and use of posters. All signs should be clear, simple and suitably visible, to direct people to the appropriate location, e.g. treatment rooms, toilets and other facilities.[25]

Bright and effective lighting systems should be provided for all indoor building areas as well as grounds around the facility and parking structures or areas. Parking for staff should be close to the building, well lit and free from heavy vegetation or anything that could conceal potential assailants. Where artificial lighting is used, ensure that it is regularly maintained to avoid flickering and failure.

Temperature should be controlled during seasonal extremes to maintain an environment that is comfortable, e.g. warm enough during the winter and cool enough during the summer, making the best use of fresh air were possible.

Client waiting rooms should be comfortable so as to avoid causing confusion, agitation, or anger. This could include: the availability of magazines, TV, fresh water, restrooms and payphones. It may also be useful to post information regarding services or other information which will help clients obtain services or more calmly wait for services. If possible, provide access to smoking areas and, where appropriate, private rooms. Adult patients and visitors can become frustrated by noisy children; likewise female patients might feel intimidated and frightened when faced with a young man who has been drinking alcohol.

Client service points such as reception desks and nurses' stations should be protected by enclosures that prevent patients from molesting, throwing objects, or reaching into the station. Such barriers should not restrict communication but protect employees.

Design of facilities should ensure uncrowded service conditions for staff.[26] Rooms for interviewing clients should ensure privacy while avoiding isolation of the staff. In emergency departments, rooms are needed in which agitated patients or family may be separated safely to protect themselves, other clients and staff. A lack of space or a poor physical layout, can create tensions between service users, this can lead to an increase in violence and aggression. Counselling or service rooms should be designed with two exits, if possible, and furniture should be arranged to prevent entrapment of staff. Doors should have unbreakable glass or plastic panels to enable colleagues to monitor the situation if there are concerns (such panels could be frosted to allow some degree of privacy). Consider the weight, size and construction of moveable objects within rooms.

Client access to staff counselling rooms, treatment rooms and other facility areas should be controlled. All doors from client waiting rooms should be locked from the inside, and outside doors locked from the outside (in accordance with fire codes) to prevent unauthorised entry. Lockable and secure bathrooms and other amenities should be provided for staff members, separate from client restrooms. All permanent and temporary employees who work in a secured area should be given keys to gain access or egress when on duty.

Allow unimpeded sight-lines with access points within sight of staff. Blind spots can make it difficult to observe patients and can lead to an increase in self-harming episodes. Curved mirrors may be installed at hallway intersections or concealed areas.

Excessive time spent waiting to be seen can sometimes lead clients to become aggressive.[27] The policy should therefore be to prevent waiting times as far as possible. Be honest about how long the person will have to wait. If you do not know how long it will be, then tell them so. Similarly, should additional delays suddenly occur, such as will happen in an emergency, explain the situation to those waiting, and tell them how long a delay is expected.

During an interview, try to prevent unwanted interruptions. Repeated interruptions of an interview either by telephone or by others coming into the room in which the nurse is seeing the client can easily unsettle some people. However, in preventing interruptions, be sure that nurses do not cut themselves off from those who might want to check on their safety.

The use of alarms

Alarm systems or panic buttons should be installed and maintained where risk is apparent or may be anticipated. Alarm systems are imperative for use in psychiatric units, hospitals, mental health clinics, emergency rooms, and where drugs are stored or dispensed. Whereas alarm systems are not necessarily preventive, they may reduce serious injury when a client is escalating in abusive behaviour.

A variety of alarm systems are available – fixed systems that are operated by panic buttons linked to the building's alarm system, personal or 'shriek' alarms. The choice of alarm system depends on the workplace, the activities undertaken, and the level of risk. Training on the use of the system is essential, as is periodic testing.

Panic button systems are hardwired systems operated by strategically placed buttons installed throughout the area where the threat exists. When they are activated, an audible or visual alarm is trigged on a monitoring console, which shows the location of the attack. One disadvantage of such systems is that unless there are a lot of buttons, a member of staff under attack may not be able to reach one before being assaulted. Because access to switches is unrestricted, patients or clients may deliberately operate them, causing false alarms. Despite this, panic buttons, where only members of staff know their location, may be useful in treatment and consulting rooms.[20]

Personal alarms may be simple 'shriek' type or may form part of more complex systems. Shriek alarms can help prevent some serious assaults. They need to be carried so that they are easy to reach in an emergency. However, a load noise may not always deter attack, and might aggravate an already potentially violent person. Such alarms are most effective in situations where other people may hear them and can respond.

CCTV

As elsewhere in Britain, CCTV is commonly in use in the public areas of hospitals. There are no special considerations required for hospitals beyond those placed by the Information Commissioner on all CCTV cameras, such as signage, registration etc. For instance it could be used to monitor the access and egress of persons coming in and going out of the hospital, to protect patients within the unit and to prevent unwelcome visitors.

Communal areas

CCTV is sometimes used in communal patient areas where the security of the service user or public safety is believed to justify this. It is central to any decision that, in line with the requirements of the Information Commissioner, a clear reason for installation is available.

Private areas

The legal basis for using CCTV in private spaces arises either from the patient's capacitated consent or because such monitoring is a proportionate response to compulsory treatment and is proportionate in an individual case.[28] This means that while it may be legal to use cameras in bedrooms, seclusion rooms and toilets, there would be a considerable burden on the provider to prove that the intrusion was proportionate. It is also arguable that the burden would be higher still if the cameras were linked to a recording device, rather than merely providing real-time unrecorded images. Very great care needs to be taken in the seating of monitors to ensure that there is no inappropriate deliberate or accidental viewing of images.

The use of CCTV is controlled by a number of statutes, regulations and guidance:[28]

- The Human Rights Act 1998
- Paragraph 16 (4) of the Private and Voluntary Health Care Regulations 2001
- The Data Protection Act 1998
- The Regulation of Investigatory Powers Act 2000
- The Mental Health Act Code of Practice
- CCTV Systems and the Data Protection Act 1998 (DPA) – guidance issued by the Information Commissioner – 2004
- Guidance issued by the NHS Security Management Service in their *NHS Security Management Manual*.

Maintenance

General maintenance must be an integral part of any safety and security systems. Prompt repair and replacement of burned out lights, broken windows or locks, etc is essential to maintain the system in safe operating condition. Delays in mending equipment, for instance broken televisions, can create tensions between patients that can lead to an increase in violence and aggression. An inability to ensure that clinical areas are maintained to an acceptable standard and that equipment is mended or replaced speedily, can impact on the morale of staff and their ability to work effectively with patients. Any mechanical device utilised for security and safety should be routinely tested for effectiveness and maintained on a scheduled basis and in accord with manufacturers' recommendations. For example, to be effective, alarm systems, including personal alarm devices, must be tested and maintained according to manufacturer and facility policy. Batteries and operation of the alarm devices should be checked by competent persons to ensure that the system functions properly.

Effective teamwork

Effective teamwork is important as it can minimise the incidence of violence and aggression by presenting a united and cohesive front.[29,30] Likewise it can promote consistency of approach and help reduce bullying and harassment. Trust within teams is essential to effective teamwork. Team members should support and encourage each other and provide sufficient time to discuss problems, feelings and worries. Having said this, conflict within teams is inevitable: not only are team members likely to have different values and beliefs, the management structures and legal frameworks under which they work are likely to differ. Conflict should not be driven underground leading to resentment, lack of trust, and ineffective work.

Conflict can become debilitating, but in moderation it is healthy; it can deepen understanding and respect, and can be diverted into creative activity. If for example, a practice nurse and a social worker conflict regarding the appropriate treatment of a client, they can manage to reach a creative compromise which is superior to either of their original ideas. This in turn, will give them confidence to cope with future conflicts and will deepen the relationship.

New team members need to feel welcome; if they do not their loyalties are likely to remain with their own professional or occupational group. New members need a period of induction and the opportunity to discuss their strengths and training needs. It is helpful if some of the information they are given is put in writing. Other team members, in turn, will need to learn the skills and potential of the newcomer. Training and induction may also be needed when someone within the team takes on a new role.

Care must be taken that people who are attached to the team, rather than being core members, are not marginalised. Their opinions should be sought and they need a congenial space in which to work. Work space is often tied to status, with those of lower status being moved around, being asked to use the corner of the desk, or having nowhere to go.

Teams typically interact with a large number of organisations, both voluntary and statutory. It is essential that a climate of goodwill is established with these organisations and that someone takes the initiative in contacting and meeting key individuals.

Roles within a team

Perhaps the most important team members, but those that are sometimes forgotten, are the patients themselves and their carers. Patients and carers need to be involved as active members of the team in order for it to function effectively. It is, for example, essential to understand patients' beliefs about health, illness and disability and to receive feedback from them in order to evaluate the service provided.

It is vitally important that team members understand and value each other's roles. This is not always easy as roles are constantly changing and role boundaries are rarely clear. This situation can, in itself, lead to uncertainty and lack of confidence, and can raise, rather than reduce, interprofessional boundaries. It is impossible to utilise the skills and experience of team members unless their roles are understood and valued. Without this understanding and respect, the team will not function at an optimum level.

Roles are rarely static and may depend on the unique composition of the team. It may, for example, be possible for the skill of diagnosing to be shared, and some aspects of the team's work, for example counselling and health education, may be undertaken by several members. Stressful tasks such as bereavement visits may also be shared.

Role negotiation is very important especially when a new member joins the team.[30] People from the same occupation or occupational group rarely have a matching set of skills and expertise, and if a team member leaves, or is away for any reason, a renegotiation of roles may be needed.

Negotiation will also be required if gaps are found between people's roles. Situations such as these can strain relationships within the best of teams, yet flexibility and the willingness to learn new skills are essential characteristics of primary healthcare workers.

Effective communication is the essence of teamwork. We have already seen that communication is vital when formulating goals and understanding other people's roles. This will be of little value, however, unless there are agreed procedures on how the tasks should be carried out and who should undertake them. Each team member must know who is responsible for implementing decisions, and someone should be nominated to see that tasks are carried through within an appropriate time scale. Many tasks are complex, and it may be helpful to break them down into smaller components. Priorities should always be set.

Protective work control systems

Organisational support and good working practices can go a long way to reducing the incidence of violence and aggression.[31,32] This includes provision of training and information as well as the reorganisation of work. There should be a consistency of approach to patient care, taking into account client concerns and requests. Changes to working practice and working hours can ensure that staff are not left alone to deal with situations that exceed both personal and professional resources. For example, there should be sufficient flexibility in staffing to identify, and adjust levels to meet security needs during patient escort, emergency responses, and meal times. There should be adequate cover for all shifts, during weekends, and during shift change. Unpredictable and unremitting workloads may lead to fatigue and a diminished ability for early identification and control of potentially violent situations. Where there is a well-established risk, there should be a trained response team which can provide transport or escort services or respond to emergencies without depleting or leaving another unit's staff at risk. Likewise, mangers should be available to assist in emergencies, provide advice, make decisions, and help with difficult individuals and situations.

Trusts should also work with local police to establish liaison and response mechanisms for police assistance and, conversely, to facilitate the hospital's assistance to local police handling emergency cases. Standard operating procedure should require the reporting of incidents of workplace violence to local police. All assaults should be investigated, reports made, and, if needed, corrective action determined.

To ensure that the policy and procedures are effective, and that the risk assessment remains valid, there should be a process of monitoring the risk control measures and reviewing the appropriateness of the policy and procedures. Unless there is senior management support and commitment, demonstrated in policy, which contains individual obligations, it is unlikely that the risk of violence will be taken seriously and controlled effectively. The policy should therefore contain an authority's statement on how the risk will be controlled. It should enable everyone to know their individual responsibilities, demonstrating the importance of involving all levels of the workforce and consulting safety representatives regarding the proposed content, implantation, monitoring, and review of policy. Management should ensure that:[33–35]

- an agreed protocol to manage risk is in operation and acted upon
- protocols for follow-up and review of patients are in place
- links with other agencies are established and maintained
- there is recognition that risk assessment and management takes time
- they provide a safe environment for their employees
- they take responsibility if need be
- training needs are assessed and appropriate support is given
- they develop good working relationships with other agencies.

Lastly, management should make available to all staff on joining the organisation, policies and guidelines relevant to the prevention, management and resolution of aggression and violence. These policies and guidelines need to be updated as necessary and adhered to.

References

1 Department of Health. *Campaign to Stop Violence against Staff Working in the NHS: NHS Zero Tolerance Zone*. Health Service Circular 1999/266. London: Department of Health.
2 Royal College of Nursing. *Working Well: a call to employers*. London: Royal College of Nursing; 2002.

3   The NHS Security Management Service (SMS). *Protecting your NHS: a professional approach to managing security in the NHS.* London: Department of Health; 2003.

4   National Institute for Mental Health (NIMHE). *Mental Health Policy Implementation Guide: developing positive practice to support the safe and therapeutic management of aggression.* London: National Institute for Mental Health; 2002.

5   Turnbull J and Paterson B (eds). *Aggression and Violence: approaches to effective management.* London: McMillan; 1999.

6   Alberg C, Bingley W, Bowers L *et al. Learning Materials on Mental Health – Risk Assessment.* Manchester: University of Manchester; 1996.

7   Bassett C. *Implementing Research in the Clinical Setting.* London: Whurr Publishing; 2001.

8   National Audit Commission. *A Safer Place to Work: protecting NHS hospital and ambulance staff from violence and aggression.* Report by the Controller and Auditor General HC527 Session 2002–03. London: The Stationery Office; 2003.

9   Vinestock M. Risk assessment: 'a word to the wise'. *Advances in Psychiatric Treatment.* 1996; **2**: 3–10.

10 Prins H. Risk assessment and management in criminal justice and psychiatry. *Journal of Forensic Psychiatry.* 1996; **7**: 42–62.

11 Royal College of Nursing. *Safer Working in the Community: a guide for NHS managers and staff on reducing the risks of violence and aggression.* London: Royal College of Nursing; 1998.

12 Lipsedge M. Clinical risk management in psychiatry. *Quality in Healthcare.* 1995; **4**: 122–8.

13 Ryan T. *Managing Crisis and Risk in Mental Health Nursing.* London: Stanley Thomas; 1999.

14 Potts J. Risk assessment and management: a Home Office perspective. In: Creighton J (ed). *Psychiatric Patient Violence: risk and response.* London: Duckworth; 1995.

15 Farrington DP. The causes and prevention of offending, with special reference to violence. In: Shepherd J (ed). *Violence in Health Care: a practical guide to coping with violence and caring for victims.* Oxford: Oxford University Press; 1994.

16 Hinde RA. Aggression at different levels of social complexity. In: Taylor PJ (ed). *Violence in Society.* London: Royal College of Physicians; 1993.

17 Pollock N, McBain I and Webster CD. Clinical decision making and the assessment of dangerousness. In: Howells K and Hollin CR (eds). *Clinical Approaches to Violence.* Chichester: John Wiley; 1989.

18 Mayhew C. *'Occupational Violence and Prevention Strategies', Master OHS and Environment Guide.* North Ryde: CCH Australia; 2003.

19 European Agency for Safety and Health at Work (EASHW). *Violence at Work.* Belgium: European Agency for Safety and Health at Work; 2002.

20 Health Development Agency. *Violence and Aggression in General Practice: guidance on assessment and management.* London: Health Development Agency; 2001.

21 Burton R. Violence and aggression in the workplace. *Mental Health Care.* 1998; **2**: 105–108.

22 Ferns T and Chojnacka I. Reporting incidents of violence and aggression towards NHS staff. *Nursing Standard.* 2005; **19**: 51–6.

23 Warshaw L and Messite J. Workplace violence: preventative and interventive strategies. *Journal of Occupational and Environmental Medicine.* 1996; **38**: 993–1005.

25 Chappell D and Di Martino V. *Violence at Work* (2e). Geneva: International Labour Office; 2000.

25 UNISON. *Violence at Work, a Guide to Risk Prevention for UNISON Branches, Stewards and Safety Representatives.* London: Unison; 1999.

26 Health Services Advisory Committee. *Violence and Aggression to Staff in Health Services: guidance on assessment and management.* Sudbury: HSE Books; 1997.

27 Bibby P. *Personal Safety for Health Care Workers*. Aldershot: Arena; 1995.

28 National Institute for Mental Health (NIMHE) *Consultation Paper on the use of CCTV*. Manchester: Manchester University; 2005.

29 Royal College of Psychiatry. *National Audit of the Management of Violence in Mental Health Settings*. Final Report Year 1. London: Royal College of Psychiatry; 2000.

30 Rowett C and Breakwell GM. *Managing Violence at Work*. Slough: Nelson; 1992.

31 Occupational Health and Safety Council. *Guidance on Workplace Violence*. London: Occupational Health and Safety Council; 2000.

32 Health and Safety Executive. *Work Related Violence*. 88/2 October 2000. London: Health and safety Executive; 2000.

33 Health and Safety Executive. *Reducing Risks – Protecting People*. London: HSE; 2004.

34 Morgan S. *Assessing and Managing Risk*. London: Pavilion; 1998.

35 Snowden P. Practical aspects of clinical risk assessment and management. *British Journal of Psychiatry*. 1997; **170**: 32–4.

Chapter 4

Managing an aggressive incident

Healthcare staff help and support people across the full spectrum of society. It is at times regrettable that staff and those that they care for come into conflict with each other. Violence and aggression can serve a number of functions and are used by different people in different ways. This puts tremendous pressure on staff as to how best to manage a situation. It can be difficult for a member of staff to respond in a professional manner when being criticised or verbally attacked for instance. However, the need to respond appropriately to the demands of the job is paramount. A good guide in structuring behaviour is that it starts and ends with self. It is important for healthcare staff to understand that they bring their own perceptions and reactions to the clinical setting. What the member of staff says and does will be scrutinised by those in their care. Patients and families, in turn, react to staff. As such, it is important that healthcare staff recognise that they are in a powerful and privileged position when dealing with clients and their relatives. Where patients are left unsupported or their needs unacknowledged, this could lead to frustrations and anger among the client population.

Recognising the risk of violence

There are times when many of us become aware of high-risk situations and are concerned for the safety of others. The possibility of violence should not be ignored or minimised but acted upon. Recognising the risk of violence is easier when you can identify the basic risk factors and the underlying motivation for violence.

It has been suggested that four elements need to be present for a violent incident to occur:[1–3]

1 *a trigger*, an event, or set of circumstances which, if present, move arousal levels towards a crisis
2 *a high level of arousal*: while arousal is not necessarily associated with violence in itself, there is a strong association between arousal, violence and aggression
3 *a weapon*, either purposely designed (knife etc), improvised (bottle, cup, etc) or anatomical (fist, teeth, etc)
4 *a target*.

Attention paid to each of these elements can help reduce the likelihood of violence occurring, both as a feature of aggression management in general, or in response to a potentially violent situation that is developing.[4] Knowledge of the patient's history and presenting complaint is likely to inform staff of likely trigger factors, which may be avoided, or the patient may be helped to resolve the issues that these trigger factors lend to their escalation.[5] Similarly, if anger or anxiety play a role in increasing the patient's emotional state, then appropriate therapeutic measures may be incorporated into the patient's treatment plan, or anger or fear may be directly addressed if they are playing a role in a particular situation.[6] Access to weapons may be controlled by monitoring the care environment and ensuring that objects that may be used for this purpose are not available, and security measures can be employed to restrict access to sharp cutlery and to prevent weapons either being brought in or manufactured. Knowledge of the characteristics of victimised patients and staff can be used to inform decisions about the appropriate placement of patients as well as the allocation of staff to particular patients and staff training and supervision.[7]

Identifying cues that warn of imminent aggression

Certain features can serve as warning signs to indicate that a person may be escalating towards physically violent behaviour.[8-10] The following list is not intended to be exhaustive and these warning signs should be considered on an individual basis.

Deterioration in general behavior and mental state

- Disorientation
- Memory impairment
- Thought processes unclear, poor concentration
- Inability to be redirected
- Inappropriate or excessive euphoria
- General over-arousal of body systems (increased breathing and heart rate, muscle twitching, dilating pupils)
- Delusions or hallucinations with violent content

Verbal aggression and threats

- Facial expressions tense and angry
- Increased volume of speech
- Prolonged eye contact
- Discontentment, refusal to communicate, withdrawal, fear, irritation
- Verbal threats or gestures
- Replicating or behaviour similar to that which preceded earlier disturbed/violent episodes
- Reporting anger or violent feelings

Changes in activity and posture

- Increased or prolonged restlessness, body tension, pacing, and excitability
- Irritability
- Extreme anxiety

Invasion of personal space

- Intrusive demands for attention
- Blocking escape routes.
- 'Eye balling'

Staff may ignore such signals because of a lack of confidence in their own skills to deal with the situation and fear that they could make matters worse rather than better. Avoidance of potential aggression is likely to increase the danger however. Consequently, an awareness of the escalation of aggression is essential. Once the danger signals are recognised, limiting action can be taken, and the probability of an early satisfactory outcome is increased.

However, staff experiences of client behaviour varies between individual workers, even in similar situations.[11] This might lead to a situation where one member of staff considers a certain behaviour as indicative of defensiveness, while another sees it as irrational behaviour. It is therefore important to be aware of the subjective and varied nature of these perceptions in assessing the behaviour of patients and their relatives. How behaviour is interpreted, the way in which it is defined, the meaning that is attached to it and the response it evokes are primarily dependent on staff perceptions. The healthcare worker who considers the expression of anger or aggression inappropriate will approach an agitated patient differently from the other who considers agitated behaviour to be meaningful.[12]

Aggressive verbal and non-verbal behaviour on the part of staff can escalate the patient's distress and violent behaviour. When staff act in a controlling manner, patients are more likely to use aggression and violence to get control. Staff who are authoritarian, disrespectful, or inflexible in their approach to patients or who have not been trained in crisis management techniques are also more likely to provoke aggressive behaviour. By recognising that people want to be involved in decisions that affect them, and play a part in their care, we as carers can begin to eliminate the frustrations that may lead to a violent incident.

It is important to note at this point that there is little conclusive evidence to suggest that violent behaviour is associated with any particular diagnosis, although some reports indicate that patients who have reduced impulse control (patients with such diagnoses as schizophrenia, bipolar disorder, organic brain syndrome, or brain injury) are at greater risk of violent episodes.

Immediate response

It is difficult to predict exactly how someone will respond when faced with the threat of violence and aggression. For many staff their choice of response could greatly determine the safety, not just of themselves, but of everyone involved, and profoundly affect their relationship with those that they care for.

The immediate response to someone escalating towards violence is to try to restore calm and stabilise their emotional state.[13] However, before this can be done an assessment of the situation needs to be made. Following this assessment, the subsequent interventions are determined by a number of seemingly competing factors:[14]

- the individual's characteristics (level of orientation, age, presenting features, diagnosis and level of risk to self and others)
- the resources available to the member of staff at the time of the incident (staffing levels and other tasks that need completing)
- the requirements of the organisation for which the individual works (particularly policies and procedures regarding the management and control of aggression and violence).

Containing an aggressive incident: the assault cycle

If the point has been reached where the potential for aggressive acts has been reached, then an assault cycle is entered. Kaplan and Wheeler describe a theoretical model that they refer to as the 'assault cycle' (*see* Figure 4.1).[15] This provides a useful analytical tool for the examination of potentially violent incidents. They describe five phases associated with incidents: (1) the trigger phase; (2) the escalation phase; (3) the crisis phase; (4) the recovery phase, and finally (5) a depression phase that occurs after the crisis. Using this five-stage model helps to identify why the aggression has occurred and the type of intervention that would be most appropriate.

The trigger phase

In this phase, as the name suggests, some event or interpersonal situation triggers an aggressive response within the individual. This could be the result of one thing or an accumulation of things. Sometimes the trigger is not obvious and the person's response seems to 'come from nowhere'. At other times, the response may seem disproportionate to the situation that the person finds themselves in and it is only through carefully questioning that we discover the true nature of the persons' complaint.

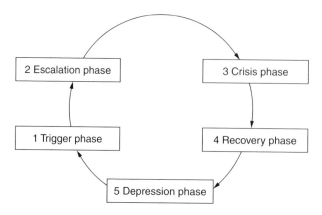

Figure 4.1 The assault cycle. Source: Kaplan and Wheeler (1983).[15]

Box 4.1   Triggers for violent incidents

- Patient actions or behaviours
- Staff action and behaviours
- Staff attitudes or approaches
- Conditions of wards
- Social environment of wards
- Communication and information to patients

Royal College of Psychiatrists (1999)[16]

The escalation phase

The person's anger and aggression begin to escalate. Stress and frustration increase. Calming measures need to be used. Feelings, emotions, attitudes, and posture all influence the way people view and listen to each other. Explaining something to someone who is feeling upset, angry, or indignant is difficult until the person's feelings have been relieved. Consequently, the person's feelings need to be recognised and acknowledged. By intervening early and disrupting the cycle of escalation, the nurse can provide a less restrictive environment where restraint and seclusion remain the last resort instead of a treatment option. A return to the previous stage is possible, and this should be the aim of interventions. However, in areas of low support, such as working in the community, the practitioner should aim to extract themselves from the situation and to return to base.

The crisis phase

Physical, emotional and psychological impulses are expressed. If escalation to the crisis stage occurs, communication is more difficult. However, if the situation becomes unsafe then personal safety and that of others in the immediate vicinity is of paramount importance. Consequently, the area around the aggressive individual should be evacuated, and help should be sought from appropriately qualified staff in sufficient numbers to safely contain the situation.

The recovery and depression phases

Agitation decreases, anxiety lessens, and communication becomes possible. At this stage, the acute crisis has ended. However, caution still needs to be maintained, as the individual may feel upset at how they have been treated and can still revert to the crisis stage. It is necessary that all staff maintain control of the situation and contain the risk of further aggression. Depending on the area, this might require the use of sedation or seclusion, in which local policies for observation will need to be implemented. Other staff that were called to help may also need to maintain their presence. Alternatively, the individual may be detained by the police.

Intervening

The first thing the staff member will have to do is make a decision as to whether they have the skills and confidence to deal with the situation, depending on the factors at play. Having made the decision to intervene it is important that the staff member lets others know what they are intending to do. In taking control of the situation the staff member will need to organise those around them, ensuring that help and support are at hand and that any instructions given are clear and concise. Where the risk is too great then do not intervene, rather alert others to the danger and make safe the area. This might mean moving other patients from the ward and calling the police.

Defusing a violent situation: de-escalation

De-escalation is defined as a resolution to a potentially violent or aggressive event by the use of empathetic alliance in a non-confrontational manner. It is a valuable intervention to help counter aggressive behaviour and if used appropriately can reduce the threat of violence.[17] It involves the use of techniques that calm down an escalating situation or service user. De-escalation is a tool that supports the ideal of 'least restrictive environment' as opposed to more restrictive measures such as chemical restraint, time out, physical restraint, and seclusion.[18] Staff should accept that in a crisis situation they are responsible for avoiding provocation. It is not realistic to expect the person exhibiting aggressive behaviour to simply calm down.

The elements of de-escalation include:[10,17,19]

- early intervention
- the use of low-arousal approaches
- identification and reduction of possible stressors and triggers
- maintaining autonomy and dignity for the patient
- provision of options and choices
- constant assessment of interventions
- avoiding physical confrontations
- provision of a safe environment.

In doing this the member of staff should:

- appear calm. The person who is angry or upset may easily perceive more hostile approaches as threatening
- approach with caution and avoid provocation wherever possible
- engage the other person in conversation, acknowledge their concerns and feelings
- use calm, respectful language, open-ended sentences, avoiding challenges and promises
- ask for facts about the problems, encourage reasoning
- ensure their own non-verbal communication is not threatening (neutral being best)
- explain their intentions to the patient and others
- maintain adequate distance

- avoid vulnerable positions and move to a place of safety. Do not put yourself in a position where you can be backed up against a wall or in a corner, and try not to back the person up against a wall, as this will only cause confrontation
- be aware of exits
- be aware of events in the immediate environment that may prolong the incident. Are others fuelling the situation by egging on the staff member or the aggressor?
- be aware of the effects of noise. Besides making it more difficult to hear, loud background noise can have a stimulating effect and increase the anger response.

Staff should also examine how they might have contributed to the patient's anger and how this might be fuelling the situation (regardless of who is at fault).

It is also worth taking into consideration any cultural factors which might explain the person's behaviour. People from different ethnic groups and cultures have very different ways of expressing emotion and may be more volatile and outspoken but pose no risk.

Where de-escalation techniques fail to sufficiently calm a situation or service user, staff should remember that verbal de-escalation is an ongoing element of the management of an escalating individual. Verbal de-escalation is supported but not replaced by appropriate physical intervention.

The healthcare worker also needs to remember they have other patients to care for and provide a safe environment for. Consequently, the healthcare worker must remain aware of how long the de-escalation process is taking and that it should preferably occur outside of the mainstream of events of the ward or unit.

As a general rule staff should:

- be supportive and avoid defensiveness. Acknowledge the existence of a problem. Accept that the patient is angry and avoid retaliatory remarks. Ask questions that focus on the aggressor
- be prepared to accept criticism. Allow the patient time to express how she or he feels and do not be in a hurry to resolve the encounter
- be reassuring in what you say and do. A warm, friendly approach with an air of quiet confidence and control will encourage the patient to feel safe. Try to match the aggressor's friendly behaviour, but meet aggressive behaviour with concern instead of anger. Show genuine concern and understanding
- use active listening skills. Remember the aggressor may have good reason to be angry, and having the full story may provide a different perspective
- avoid situations where the aggressor may fear loss of face through backing down. Not wanting to look like a loser may turn the encounter into a fight. Make it easy for the patient to back down. Always be prepared to offer a compromise. Do not offer too submissive a response however, as this may make the patient even angrier if they do not feel an attempt is being made to understand their needs. Being passive is also unhelpful, and could incite aggression as the patient strives to elicit a response.

Responding to an aggressive person

When responding to the needs of an aggressive person it is important to try and restore calm and bring a measure of control to the situation in order to bring about a more rational appraisal of what is happening. Good communication skills are an essential part of this process and are a key factor in the management and prevention of violence and aggression.[20–22] It is through communication that helping relationships are formed, problems are identified and discussed, and information is conveyed.

There are two aspects to communication, verbal and non-verbal. Verbal communication is principally achieved through the spoken word, including the underlying emotion, context and connotation of what is actually said.[23] It can be used to convey information accurately and efficiently. However, it is a less effective means of communicating feelings or nuances of meaning, and it represents only a small segment of total human communication.

People will often assume that they are on the same 'wavelength' when talking to each other, however this is not always the case. Because words are only symbols, they seldom mean precisely the same thing to two people If the word represents an abstract idea such as 'depressed' or 'hurt', the chance of mis-understanding or misinterpretation may be great particularly in a heightened situation. That is why it is important for staff to listen carefully to what the person has to say by checking their interpretation and incorporating information from the non-verbal level as well.

Problem solving

When the situation is calmer, encourage the individual to identify and explain the nature of the problem, and to try and identify a solution.[24] Do not agree or disagree and be careful not to get drawn into an argument, or to promise anything that cannot be delivered, as this could escalate the situation. This is a useful method of getting the person to take responsibility for their actions by promoting a sense of ownership and control over the situation, especially if you can get them to identify the best and most appropriate way forward.

Certain phrases may be provocative and make an aggressive individual even angrier. Examples include: 'Now don't be silly', 'Pull yourself together', 'This is no way for an adult to behave', or even, 'You're not the only person with this problem!'. While the latter might seem an obvious thing not to do, it is surprising how many times the author has heard such phrases used in clini-cal practice, particularly where the staff member has been under pressure or feeling threatened.

Information giving

Information giving is a fundamental part of the healthcare workers' role, to the point that its importance is sometimes forgotten. Patients and their relatives can become agitated and threaten to harm staff when information is not forthcoming or is withheld.[25] Confusion as to what is expected of the patient and not being involved in decisions relating to their care can provoke similar responses. The healthcare worker can determine what the patient's information needs are by asking questions and employing empathy. When giving information, it is best to give important messages first in order that they are understood and retained. Repeating and stressing points is another strategy by which information is taken on board. Also, try to be consistent in what you are saying and avoid confusing and conflicting messages.

Validation

Often, people who experience intense anger and rage feel isolated and may view themselves as alone in having these feelings.[26] The healthcare worker can use past experience and knowledge to normalise the patient's reaction and validate the experience, and in turn bring control to the situation. For example, it may be appropriate to give the person 'permission' to use foul language as a means of expressing themselves, acknowledging that it is something you do when angry or frustrated.

Depersonalising the situation

Depersonalise the issues in circumstances where you have no personal influence over decisions, refusing requests etc. Let the person know it is not your personal decision, but is due to the policy of the organisation. Provide information about complaint procedures and alternative sources of help, if appropriate.

Personalising the situation

This is the opposite of the above, where you take responsibility for your actions and decisions in an effort to promote dialogue and understanding of the matter. In doing so it allows the two of you to explore alternatives and engage on a much more personal level.

Exploring beliefs

It can be useful to explore the beliefs the patient has about the expression of anger.[27] Discussion of beliefs that prevent the person from seeking alternative ways of handling the situation may help the patient to take charge of the situation. Interventions of this kind are designed to help the person in finding alternatives to the use of violence and aggression, and should be encouraged.

Listening to the patient's illness experience

Often patients and their family members are invited to provide details about past medical treatments, medication, hospitalisations, and therapies. What is overlooked is the experience of the health problem or the experience of inter-actions with professionals. Inviting patients and their families to talk about their previous experiences with the healthcare system may highlight both their concerns and resources.

Praising

For praise to be effective it needs to be given with respect at a time that is both appropriate and in keeping with the situation. A commendation is a 'statement of special praise that is specific to some aspect of the patient and/or family functioning'.[26] A commendation focuses on the patient's behaviour across time and highlights the patient's strengths and resources. Often in clinical settings the focus becomes 'problem saturated' and what the patient does well is overlooked. For example, commending a person's decision to remove themselves from an over-stimulating environment highlights their ability to assume control and take responsibility for thoughts and feelings that may have previously invited aggressive behaviour.

Rewarding

Appropriate and sustained progress by the patient in tackling their aggression should be rewarded. This could be in the form of a tangible reward such as being allowed off the ward or increased staff time. In this way it is demonstrated to the patient that it is the behaviour and not the person that is under scrutiny.

Providing choices

Whenever possible, the healthcare worker should provide the patient with choices, particularly patients who have little control over their situation because of their condition. For example the patient who is experiencing a manic episode and confined to her room may have few options over her daily schedule.

Jargon

Every professional and occupation group has its jargon and the health professions are certainly no exception.[28] It is a common mistake to use medical and organisational jargon when questioning and communicating information to patients. The patient may not understand these terms, which can lead to embarrassment. Care must be taken to avoid jargon, but at the same time, it is important not to be patronising as people are now exposed to a great deal of health-related information through the media. By carefully explaining technical terms, the health worker also has an opportunity to provided patients with information that they may encounter in other contexts. Healthcare workers should attempt to gauge the patient's verbal ability and adjust the content of their speech accordingly. Patients have their own jargon when attempting to describe the signs and symptoms of illness. Examples are 'I feel low' or 'I feel funny'. It is important that health workers do not take patient's jargon at face value, but rather try to clarify what they mean. Pain is another good example of patient jargon, and it is important to identify the degree of pain the person is in and how they are coping with it.

Talking to an aggressive person: non-verbal communication

Every time verbal communication takes place it is complemented with a complex repertoire of movements and gestures.[23] They are usually congruous to the verbal message but sometimes they may be conflicting. Non-verbal communication is often unconsciously motivated and may more accurately indicate a person's meaning than the words being spoken. It helps to maintain the flow of communication and acts as a subtle indicator to show when a person has finished speaking. By observing the patient's gait, posture, and facial expression, the healthcare worker can learn a great deal about the way the person is feeling and their possible intentions. If non-verbal signals and words conflict, the non-verbal signals may give a stronger impression than the words, although the overall message may be confusing.

Non-verbal communication can distort verbal information as well as enhance it. Lack of facial expression or a monotonous voice, for instance, may act as a barrier to communication. Some non-verbal communication cannot be changed: for example, age, race, sex and physical appearance. A person's accent is another relatively stable characteristic by which people are often evaluated. There is a tendency to make global inferences about people on the basis of very limited information, and to minimise just how much people's behaviour is affected by the situation and environment they are in, especially if they perceive it as strange or intimidating.[29]

Not only is it important to be sensitive to the person's non-verbal communication, but sensitivity to and awareness of our own body signals is also vital.[30] Using body language appropriately in a helping relationship can help to facilitate a client's trust and confidence in the healthcare worker. The use of tone of voice, eye contact, touch, facial expression and posture can convey qualities of genuineness and warmth. Using non-verbal communication effectively can relax the client and increase the likelihood of them exploring their problems in a more constructive manner. In turn, the more relaxed patients feel, the more likely they are to exhibit their usual behaviour.

Healthcare workers may influence what patients say and how they behave, not only by what they say, but also by their non-verbal communication and use of silence. If healthcare workers only respond positively when patients mention improvement of symptoms, for example, patients may become inhibited about admitting that the condition is static or worsening.

Even when we are silent we communicate a lot – through our eyes, facial expression, posture, gestures and personal appearance. Through these non-verbal behaviours we communicate who we are and how we feel. Others draw conclusions about our sincerity, credibility and emotional state based on our non-verbal behaviour. Poor eye contact, slouching, nervous gestures and other non-assertive behaviours can convince others that what we have to say can be safely ignored.

Types of non-verbal behaviours

There are various types of non-verbal behaviours. Each of these is greatly influenced by the social and cultural background of the person. *Vocal cues* or *paralinguistic cues* include all the non-verbal qualities of speech.[23] Some examples include pitch, tone of voice, quality of voice, loudness or intensity, rate and rhythm of talking, and unrelated non-verbal sounds such as laughing, groaning and nervous coughing, and sounds of hesitation. These are particularly vital cues of emotion and can be powerful conveyors of information. The most important of these and the easiest to control are loudness and speed. Nervousness can make us speak too softly to be heard, or so loudly that we distract from our message. Speak loudly and slowly enough to be heard and understood. It is also important to control how you end your sentences. Raising the pitch of your voice at the end of a sentence makes the sentence sound like question. A slight lowering of pitch at the end of a sentence makes it sound like a statement.

Activity 4.1

The meaning behind words is conveyed in the way in which they are spoken. Consider how you use the following when communicating with those that you care for:

- clarity of voice
- volume
- tone of voice
- silence
- speed at which you speak.

Action cues are body movements, sometimes referred to as *kinetics*.[23] They include automatic reflexes, posture, facial expression, gestures, mannerisms, and actions of any kind. Facial movements and posture can be particularly significant in interpreting the speaker's mood. Our face tells others the degree to which we are alert, interested, in agreement, or relaxed. It reveals the types of emotions we feel. It is best to keep your facial expression as neutral as possible when engaged with an aggressive patient.

Object cues are the speaker's intentional and non-intentional use of all objects.[23] Dress, furnishings and possessions all communicate something to the observer about the speaker's sense of self. These cues often are consciously selected by the individual however, and therefore may be chosen to convey a certain look or meaning. Thus they can be less accurate than other types of non-verbal communication. Uniforms give information regarding occupation and status and may engender feelings of respect, fear, or trust, or create a psychological distance between the healthcare worker and the patient.

Touch is possibly the most personal of the non-verbal messages. A person's response to it is influenced by setting, cultural background, type of relationship, sex of communicators, ages, and expectations. Its use can express a striving to connect with another person as a way of meeting them or relating to them. Likewise, it can be a way of expressing or conveying something to another, such as concern, empathy, or caring. Touch can also be used receptively as a way of sensing, perceiving, or allowing signalling of our intent; however it can also be intrusive in some intimate procedures of healthcare. Touch in the common course of treatment can be a sign of positive communication; aggression is also primarily expressed through bodily contact and therefore it is recommended to avoid touching clients who are aroused or angry.

> **Box 4.2** Non-verbal channels of communication
>
> - *Bodily behaviour*: posture, body movements, and gestures
> - *Facial expressions*: snarling, frowns, raised eyebrows and turning down of the mouth
> - *Voice-related behaviour*: tone of voice, pitch, voice level, intensity, spacing of words, emphasis, pauses, silences and fluency
> - *Observable automatic physiological responses*: quickened breathing, the development of a temporary rash, blushing, paleness and pupil dilation
> - *Physical characteristics*: fitness, height, weight and complexion
> - *General appearance*: grooming and dress

Eye contact

Eye contact is also an important and sometimes misunderstood area of engagement.[31] In an escalating aggressive situation there are various types of exchange:

- *stage 1* is before any aggressive interaction has taken place and the eye contact is of an ordinary pattern
- *stage 2* is where either or both parties sense that the conversation is gradually becoming more heated, and one or both attempt to minimise eye contact
- *stage 3* is where the situation is unambiguously aggressive and almost out of hand. This is where eye contact is of a long duration, high intensity, challenging and aversive.

The task therefore, is to try to maintain the pattern of ordinary eye contact, appropriate to stage 1, apparently not noticing any changes in eye contact demonstrated by the other person. If eye contact is too threatening, however, averting the gaze to the shoulders is effective as it signifies non-confrontational interest, but it also allows the aggressor to be kept in full view at all times.

Posture

The moment you walk into a room, your posture and carriage communicate messages about your confidence, how you expect to relate to others, your energy level and emotional state. Slouching may say 'Don't notice me', or 'I'm tired and can be easily worn down', or 'I'm not interested in being here'. Slouching does not invite the other to take you seriously. A tense and rigid posture communicates you are in a heightened emotional state. It may be interpreted as anxiety or anger depending on your other non-verbal behaviours. This kind of posture makes you look out of control. An erect and relaxed posture while standing and sitting communicates confidence, self-control, energy and an expectation that you are to be taken seriously. When sitting, leaning forward slightly communicates interest and a sense of purpose. Leaning back communicates disinterest or disagreement. Crossing your arms and legs suggests a tense and closed attitude, while uncrossed arms and legs suggest a relaxed and open attitude.

Gestures

Gestures can be used to accentuate and support your message or to distract and discredit. Nervous fidgeting and tense jerky movements are distracting. These types of gestures and movements make you look out of control and seriously diminish your persuasive power. If you have trouble controlling nervous and fidgety movements, channel your nervous energy by taking notes. Hand and arm movements can be used to emphasise what you say. Do not emphasise everything, however. Be judicious in your use of gestures. Keep your gestures relaxed, fluid and moderate in size. Gestures which are too large make you look grandiose, while gestures which are too small make you look nervous.

Boundaries

Healthcare workers play an active role not only in the treatment and support of patients, but also in setting limits and defining boundaries.[32] The boundaries of the staff–patient relationship are defined by the roles of the staff and patient. It is the staff's responsibility to define the boundaries because, in many instances, circumstances prevent the patient from being able to define them accurately. Professional relationship boundaries are complex and sometimes unclear. Because the patient is asked to share information usually reserved only for intimate relationships, the patient becomes vulnerable and dependent on those about them. The vulnerability and the dependency place the power of the relationship in the hands of the nurse. It is the nurse's responsibility to be clear about relationship limits to protect the integrity of the person. If a staff member attempts to meet personal needs through a patient relationship, then professional boundaries are violated. When professional boundaries are violated, the relationship shifts into a non-therapeutic one. Boundary violations can lead to an escalation of the violent situation. In practice, roles cannot easily be compartmentalised as they have elaborate interconnections with each other. Some of the behaviour demonstrated in the role of a friend may be replicated in the role of the healthcare worker. Although some of the behaviour expected in one role may be complementary to another, there may be circumstances when roles are in tension, for instance, it might be unwise to reveal things of a personal nature to the patient.

Body zones

Every individual is surrounded by four different body zones that provide varying degrees of protection against unwanted physical closures during interactions with others.[26,27] The first zone, the immediate zone, as it is called, surrounds and protects an individual from others. Only persons with whom an individual has an immediate relationship (e.g. spouse or parent) can voluntarily enter this zone. If anyone else attempts to enter, the individual will move to protect the space. This they can do in a number of ways, from moving back from the other person, to ignoring them completely. The individual who cannot protect the immediate zone becomes anxious and may become aggressive. The next area, the personal zone, begins at the boundary of the immediate zone and ends at the social zone.

People who have personal relationships with the individual, such as friends or family members, can comfortably enter this zone and be received. A healthcare worker can enter the zone during the establishment of a relationship. The social zone extends outward from the border of the personal zone to the public zone. Acquaintances and strangers can comfortably interact with the individual in the social zone. In the most distant boundary the public zone, there is little meaningful interaction, but it can be used for reorganising and acknowledging the presence of another.

The actual size of the different zones varies according to culture. Some cultures define the immediate zone narrowly and the personal zones widely. Thus, friends in these cultures stand and sit close to each other while interacting. Other cultures define the immediate zone widely and are uncomfortable when people stand close to them. The variability of immediate and personal zones has implications for staff. For a patient to be comfortable with the healthcare worker, the immediate zone of that individual needs protected. Care staff will usually be allowed to enter the personal zone, but the patient will express discomfort if the immediate zone is breached. For the care worker the difficulty lies in differentiating the personal zone from the immediate zone for each patient.

The healthcare worker's awareness of his or her own need for immediate and personal space is another prerequisite for therapeutic intervention with the patient. It is important that a nurse feels comfortable while interacting with patients. Establishing a comfort zone may well entail fine-tuning of the size of body zones. Recognising this will help nurses understand their sometimes inexplicable reactions to proximity of patients. The general rule is that if it does not feel comfortable for either party, staff or patient, then there is the need to move back and possibly try a different type of approach.

Intrusiveness

Another intervention that may precede violence by patients might be called intrusiveness or perceived attack. In this case, the patient or client becomes aggressive because they perceive some sort of verbal or physical attack is being made upon them by staff, for example a confused patient may mistake an offer of help in adjusting an item of clothing as an assault on their person.[33] Actual attacks on patients by staff are rare but not unknown. However, the emphasis here is on the patient's perception or appraisal of the staff behaviour. Verbal attack may be perceived if staff insult, threaten, or otherwise reject the patient.

Physical intrusiveness is an even greater problem since much of the care delivered by health staff inevitably involves physical contact with patients. Patients may perceive staff that simply approach them and encroach on their personal space as making some form of attack upon them, and they may be particularly prone to such perceptions when distressed (or in a state of confusion). This is why it is important to communicate your intentions to the patient and seek their consent to intervene.

In addition, some healthcare procedures are more likely to be perceived as an attack because they actually result in pain for the patient (e.g. giving an injection). It is clearly important therefore that patients are informed of the nature of the procedure, to enable them to appraise the interaction more appropriately, and that their consent is obtained where possible prior to physically intruding in this way.

Interviewing

Interviewing patients is an important aspect of assessment and an ongoing process throughout treatment. It is a potential flashpoint for aggression, and therefore worth consideration here.[34] Effective clinical interviewing is dependent on a variety of interpersonal skills, which include proficiency in asking questions, the ability and motivation to listen and respond sensitively, and the capacity to understand and emit non-verbal cues. The acquisition of these skills in clinical education and practice has tended to be taken for granted and thought to be largely a matter of common sense. Lack of skill in this area can, however, have far-reaching negative consequences in terms of patient satisfaction and compliance with advice.

Types of interview

There are many types of interview, ranging from those that are highly structured to the very unstructured type. In structured interviews, very specific questions are asked which can be coded easily, often by means of a standard chart or form. Conversely, with an unstructured interview there is little attempt to formulate the content, which is written out in full. Most interviews conducted by healthcare workers fall somewhere between the two extremes and are said to be semi-structured.

There are advantages and disadvantages to both structured and unstructured interviews; a highly structured interview may run counter to an ideology of free expression or an holistic approach to patient care, and may be inappropriate for certain patients, for example young children, or people with complex problems. On the other hand, some patients may regard an open-ended, holistic approach as an invasion of privacy.

The main advantages of the structured interview are that patients' responses can be categorised and coded relatively easily, irrelevant information can be avoided, and timing can be kept under control. There is the danger, however, of assuming that structured information is more factual and reliable than it really is.

In order to gain relevant information, the health worker's questions are selective and focused. This may lead to interesting and relevant information falling outside of the health worker's frame of reference to be lost. Morrall believes that, in order for a consultation to be successful the healthcare worker and the patient must share understanding of the problem.[35] If the interview is highly structured, the health worker's definition is likely to dominate.

There is a danger with the structured approach, particularly with inexperienced staff, that the exercise of filling in the assessment form correctly over-rides the importance of the patient/health worker relationship, with considerable therapeutic effects. The health worker may become preoccupied with the mechanisms of recording the interview data, or frustrated if the patient's responses are vague or confused. There is a tendency for people to develop rigid routines over time, whereby they adhere strictly to a given assessment format without considering its usefulness to the particular patient concerned.

Most writers on the subject of clinical interviewing advocate a relatively unstructured approach. Hindle believes that health workers should avoid over-controlling patients, or they may feel intimidated and relevant information may be lost.[36] They believe that health workers should listen more than talk. The traditional training of health workers has tended to emphasise the need to be 'doing something'.[37] Helping is not necessarily dependent on talking or doing, and the healthcare worker should steer clear of taking refuge in care activities in order to avoid listening to patients.

It is also worth mentioning at this point a phenomenon known as the social desirability effect. This refers to the tendency people have to present themselves in a favourable light, a process which Goffman referred to as 'impression management'.[38] Patients may feel that various aspects of their lives will discredit them in the eyes of the health worker, for example unemployment, lack of hygiene, or habits and addictions such as smoking and alcoholism. Patients are unlikely to disclose discrediting information to the health worker unless an empathetic atmosphere, free from anxiety and moral evaluations, can be created. This may be particularly so with people suffering mental health problems, which are still stigmatised in our society, leading to feelings of shame and inadequacy and at times anger and frustration.

Watkins suggests the following factors that may become barriers in engaging with patients:[39]

- secret agendas: not being honest with the patient, not putting the client first
- inflexibility of context: the nurse's reluctance to be flexible in where to meet a client in the community
- fears of intimacy: a nurse's own issues, their personal history, feeling vulnerable/inexperienced due to previous contact with clients
- insensitivity to race, culture, gender, values, beliefs
- using previous history and making assumptions about a client
- personal beliefs and prejudices about mental illness
- making sweeping generalisations and judgements about clients and their needs.

Questioning

In order to help someone there is a need to find out what is troubling them. Sensitivity on the part of staff to the questions they ask can help reduce the incidence of violence and aggression. A useful guideline is to use open questions which provoke thought, rather than direct or closed questions, which may produce yes or no answers.[37] An example of a closed question is 'Are you feeling better or worse?'. This makes categorisation of the response easy but the information gained is minimal. An alternative open question would be 'Please will you describe how you feel?'. The reply may be complex, rambling, and difficult to categorise, but nonetheless full and rich. Closed questions are, however, useful for gathering factual information.[37] They are easy to answer and provide clarity and focus. Open questions are useful for opening up conversation and providing clues to what is troubling the patient. It should also be appreciated that some patients are not sufficiently articulate to cope with open questions.

Leading questions

Leading questions influence the direction of the patient's reply and, as a general rule, should be avoided. For example, the question, 'How did you find the medication?' makes the assumption that the patient took it. This may, in turn, lead to an unwillingness on the part of the patient to admit that the medication was not taken but discarded.

Loaded questions

Loaded questions are those which are emotionally coloured giving rise to a feeling of approval or disproval. An example is, 'I hope you haven't forgotten to take your medication today!'. The healthcare worker is expressing a judgement requiring what the patient should or ought to do. Questions which are loaded with moral judgements and evaluations should generally be avoided as the patient is likely to respond to the emotional rather than the factual content. It is not always easy to avoid such questions however, because what is regarded as judgemental by one person may be viewed as neutral by another.

Multiple questions

Multiple questions require two or more answers. An example of a multiple question is 'Are you feeling angry or frightened at the moment?'. Questions requiring two or more responses should be avoided as they are difficult to answer and confusing to both patients and healthcare workers.

The wording and ordering of questions

The wording and ordering of questions is also important and needs a great deal of care. Even small changes in wording can bring about large changes in response and therefore require attention and thought. On most occasions it is best to begin an interview by asking for factual information of a neutral kind. When rapport has been established, patients are more likely to feel comfortable and respond to more intimate questioning. Do not ask too many questions, and always listen for the client's reply. It should be noted, however, that even simple demographic questions may be viewed by some people as intimate, for example asking for details of age or ethnic origin.

Sometimes patients are only too keen to explain particular aspects of their problems to healthcare workers, and this is to be encouraged particularly when seeking to calm someone. It may also enable healthcare workers to gain insight into how patients view their illness and experience of receiving care.

Help them to talk in more specific terms by focusing on what they say and asking for clarification. Support them by repeating key words or phases. These indicate that you have heard what they have to say, and encourage the client to express underlying fear, anxieties or uncertainties.

Questions of any kind will only produce accurate information if they are understood by the client. Therefore they must be clearly stated and unambiguous. Try to avoid questions which begin with why? People often do not know why they feel or experience situations in a specific way. The good use of questions should help the client understand themselves more clearly and realistically.

Active listening

The way in which we listen (or fail to listen) can be a major barrier in our interpersonal relationships. If we are to fully understand, we need to learn to listen effectively. We need to listen not only to words, but also to the hidden feelings and intentions that are expressed.

It is also vital that the health worker clarifies the patient's complaint. This means listening to what he or she is saying and making sure the reasons for the consultation are clear. Verbal and non-verbal clues are important and may be missed if full attention is not given to the patient. Active listening focuses on what the patient is saying, to enable the healthcare worker to respond to the message in an objective manner. While listening, the healthcare worker concentrates only on what the patient is saying and the underlying meaning. The healthcare worker's verbal and non-verbal behaviour indicates active listening. The healthcare worker usually responds indirectly using techniques such as open-ended statements, reflection, and questions that elicit additional responses from the patient. In active listening, the healthcare worker should avoid changing the subject, and instead follow the lead of the patient. However, at times it is necessary to respond directly by using techniques such as questions to help a patient focus on a specific topic. As we listen, we attempt to make sense of, retain and judge what the speaker is saying. We plan what we are going to say in response, and we covertly rehearse our response.[36]

You can test whether or not you have understood the other party by summarising your understanding of what was said and asking for verification. This not only lets you know whether you have understood the other correctly, it also lets the other person know they have been understood. Some problem-solving or negotiation sessions get stuck because people do not realise that they understand one another. Many times the issue is not confusion, but disagreement about what to do about the problem. Working out solutions is different from establishing an understanding, and some issues remain unresolved because parties never get past the stage of establishing that all viewpoints are understood. Examples of blocks to listening are shown in Box 4.3.

Box 4.3 Blocks to listening

- *Comparing*: 'What's he complaining about, there's a lot more patients worse off than him?'
- *Mind reading*: trying to figure out what the other person is thinking and feeling

- *Rehearsing*: giving attention to the preparation and delivery of your next comment
- *Filtering*: listening to some things and not to others
- *Judging*: not listening to what they have to say, as you have already judged them
- *Dreaming*: half-listening while something the other person says triggers off a chain of associations of your own
- *Identifying*: referring everything the other person says to our own experience
- *Advising*: being the great problem solver; offering advice where it is not wanted
- *Sparring*: arguing and debating. You disagree so quickly that the other person never feels heard. You take strong stands and are clear about your beliefs, values and preferences
- *Being right*: going to any lengths to avoid being wrong
- *Derailing*: changing the subject suddenly
- *Placating*: this is where you agree with everything and do not really listen to what is being said

Adapted from McKay *et al.* (1983).[40]

Finally, today more than ever before, staff need to be prepared to communicate effectively with people from a variety of ethno-cultural backgrounds. The healthcare worker–patient relationship may be hampered by a lack of under-standing and use of common language. Patients may even revert to their native tongue as a means of not engaging with staff. In using verbal communication sensitively as a tool to promote mutual respect based on understanding and acceptance of cultural differences, the healthcare worker may go some way to bridging this gap. The healthcare worker may also communicate respect for the patient's dialect by adapting to the patient's linguistic style and using fewer words, more gestures, or more expressive facial behaviours.

Further responses to an aggressive person

The following section will examine a range of strategies used in managing violence and aggression, some of which can be used in the immediacy of the situation, and others can be used over a longer time period.

Mood matching

This is where the arousal level is matched between all people in the interaction. For example, in a conversation with someone who is depressed, people attempt to be slightly 'downbeat'. Similarly, the mood is reasonably cheerful when talking to someone who is happy or excited about something.

In contrast, when talking to somebody who is agitated, people attempt to be calm, so as not to inflame the situation. The danger of this is that it can be misinterpreted as indifference. One option is to match the other person with a similar level of energy. However, in this instance, energy would not be displayed as aggression; rather it would be shown by concern, involvement, and interest.

Mirroring

This is the physical equivalent of mood matching. Mirroring is exactly as it says: it is where one person physically reflects the way the other person is sitting or standing. Normally this occurs entirely spontaneously; if one person sits back then so does the other one, if one person comes forward then the other does likewise, and so forth. Observational research shows that people who are mirroring each other tend to get on better than those who do not ('getting on' being measured by the length of the conversation they have), in spite of the fact that this is normally going on unconsciously. It is possible to utilise this phenomenon to enhance the interactions with the aggressor. This needs to be done with some caution, however, as, if exaggerated, it may be seen to be mimicking or mocking.

Interrupting patterns

Although the patients are not usually aware of it, escalation of feelings, thoughts and behaviour from calmness to violence usually follow a particular pattern. Disruption of the pattern can sometimes be a useful means of preventing escalation, and can help the patient regain composure. A number of strategies can be used to interrupt patterns, for example, distraction, diversion, and thought stopping.

Distraction

Efforts are made to distract the patient from escalating aggression by engaging them in activity more to their liking, such as gong for a walk or listening to their favourite music.

Diversion

Diversion is similar to distraction, except that efforts are made to address the source of the person's anger once a sense of calm has returned. This is con-sidered more productive than just 'blanking out' the problem, as it provides the means to explore new ideas, opinions, information, or education about a particular problem.

Thought stopping

The patient is asked to identify thoughts that heighten feelings of anger and is invited to 'turn the thoughts off' by focusing on other thoughts and activities. For example, 'counting to ten', reciting the words of a favourite song, preparing the next day's shopping list.

Anticipation of needs

It is important in clinical assessment to consider the environment as it may be seen from the patient's view. Coming into hospital can be confusing, and it is up to staff to aid the patient in adjusting to their new situation. A lack of understanding as to what is required of the patient and ward routine can increase feelings of insecurity and lead to possible aggression. Appropriate interventions include clarifying the meaning and purpose of persons and objects in the environment, reducing the amount of information the patient needs to take on board, reducing stimuli wherever possible, and explaining rules and procedures.

Reduction in stimulation

For persons whose perceptions or thoughts are disordered from brain damage, degeneration, or other thought-processing difficulties, modification of the environment may be one of the main interventions of choice. It has been suggested that people differ as to the level of stimulation they need or prefer. Normally, people adjust their environments accordingly, for example, some people like their music loud, whereas others like it soft; some people prefer to deal with their problems on their own, whereas others seek the support and company of staff.

Within a disordered brain or an unusually restrictive environment, those adjustments may not be within the person's control. The person with brain injury, progressive dementia, or distorted vision may be experiencing intense and highly confusing stimulation, even though from the healthcare worker's or family's perspective, all seems calm and orderly. The healthcare worker can make stimuli meaningful, or simplify and interpret the environment in many practical ways. Some examples are identifying people or equipment that may be unfamiliar, providing clues as to what is expected (e.g. posting signs with directions, putting toothbrush and toothpaste by the sink), removing or silencing unnecessary stimuli (e.g. turning off paging systems, which can be startling to patients).

Often, cognitively impaired patients exhibit repetitive behaviours such as wandering and making noises. These actions may be the patient's means of remaining connected to their environment, and attempts to interrupt them may lead to the patient striking out. Engaging the patient in a simple exercise, such as playing catch or moving to music, may help reduce this type of behaviour. Other actions that can be taken include providing structured activities that use previously learned motor skills.

Communicating assertively

Farrell and Gray make the observation that being assertive is an effective way of dealing with aggression.[41] The word assertiveness is used to describe a certain kind of behaviour which helps us to communicate clearly and confidently our needs, wants and feelings to other people, without abusing in any way their human rights. It is an alternative to passive, aggressive and manipulative behaviour.

The application of assertiveness in situations that threaten aggression assumes that people are attacked or victimised, or are in danger of becoming aggressive themselves, partly because they do not express their wishes, or do so in a socially ineffective manner.[42] While assertiveness training may help people who are not confident to manage difficult situations more effectively, there are those that this approach does not suit, and who are not comfortable with being assertive.

Like any skill, assertive behaviour must be learnt, practised and refined. Sometimes people do not get the opportunity to learn appropriate assertive behaviour. In other circumstances that behaviour is not reinforced through practice, and can be replaced by other less healthy styles of interaction. At other times people may not feel they have a legitimate right to act assertively. In some instances a bad experience or succession of events can undermine a person's belief in their right to be assertive, and they can find themselves acting in a passive fashion.

Box 4.4 gives some techniques that can be helpful in promoting an assertive approach. A hallmark of practising being assertive is making 'I' statements. 'I' statements cause a person to take responsibility for their feelings, ideas and needs. By adopting such an approach it means coming to the realisation that you cannot change other people's behaviours. You can only change your response and/or communicate what you need. This is not to say that you will always be successful in changing the behaviour of others. First of all, it is not up to someone else to meet your needs. The important thing is that you are more likely to be respected, taken seriously and get more of what you want. An important point here is that of compromise. Sometimes in order to get what you want you have to give up something in return.

Box 4.4   Types of assertion

Different types of assertive statements are available to you. They are:

- *simple assertion*: 'I want you to take this four times a day, every day, until they're completely gone'
- *empathic assertion*: 'I can tell that having to take three different medicines seems overwhelming to you right now'
- *confrontive assertion*: 'I can see that you are a busy person, but I really need to talk to you about your medication'
- *negative feeling assertion*: 'I feel really frustrated when I have trouble explaining to you how to properly take your medicine. You seem to feel that this is your wife's responsibility more than your own'
- *positive feeling assertion*: 'I really like it that you come in on the exact day that you are scheduled for your refill'

Broken record

You may find yourself in a situation where you are trying to make a point, but the other person seems to be ignoring your request, or maybe showing refusal. The other person may be continually trying to distract you with different issues. Choose a phrase with which you feel comfortable and, without getting angry or shouting, repeat the original assertive statement each time the person tries to divert you or asks you to change your mind. Resist the temptation to justify, answer or get angry. For example, 'In my professional opinion, it is not advisable for you to drink alcohol while taking medication' (repeated to the individual as often as required).

Workable compromise

If you find that the broken record technique has not worked, it is useful to follow with a compromise. The main thing is to ensure that you maintain your self-respect, not that you get your own way.

Fogging

If we are criticised – even unfairly – we often develop feelings of guilt and insecurity. When this happens we may become defensive and begin to make excuses. Alternatively we may involve ourselves in an argument that gets us nowhere.

Fogging can be used to deal with criticism which is invalid. It affords us a means to deal with people who try to influence us to behave in a certain way by means of criticising us unjustly. By using it we can create a situation which makes it impossible for them to have any success. By acknowledging to the critic that there may be some truth in what they are saying (as they see it) you will remain in charge of what you decide to do.

Some tips:

- do not deny the criticism (provides more ammunition)
- do not become defensive (admitting the criticism may be justified)
- do not counter-criticise (starts an argument)
- listen to exactly what the critic is saying – respond using the same words
- Respond only to what is said – not to what is being implied.

Negative assertion

This technique allows you to admit to making an error without 'crawling'. Conditioning in our childhood has often created the belief within us that what we should feel guilty when we make mistakes. Most of us need to work on ourselves to allow us to cope with errors and criticisms. Negative assertion is just that, e.g.

- 'Yes, I'm afraid that this is my work, and yes it is wrong. I will re-do it straight away'
- 'Yes, I am sorry. It is rather messy. You are quite right'

Sorting issues

Occasionally, in the course of an interaction, several issues will become sandwiched together. Unless these messages are sorted out and dealt with separately, the individual may begin to feel confused, anxious and guilty. Thus, it is to both parties' advantage to deal with these different issues separately.

Selective ignoring

Selective ignoring is the discriminatory attending and non-attending of specific content from another individual. Replies are not given to unfair or abusive interaction, but instead only to statements that are not destructive, guilt-provoking, prejudicial, or unjust.

Disarming anger

Disarming anger can be an extremely useful protective technique. It involves an honest contract offered to another individual who is exhibiting high amounts of anger and who may, in fact, be bordering on physical violence. The contract tries to work out an agreement, stating that you will talk about whatever issue the other person wants, but only after some of the anger dissipates. Writing down an angry person's comments will often help to diffuse his or her anger. It also slows the person down because you cannot write as fast as the person can yell. Further, when a record is being kept, an individual will frequently choose his or her words more cautiously. However, in writing things down, observation of the person may be diminished and therefore you might be more open to attack.

Saying no

Try saying no when you want to refuse a request. Try to say no without feeling guilty or expressing an apology. Many people feel unhappy when refusing a request in an assertive way, feeling that it somehow means they are rejecting the person. Using empathy softens the no, e.g. 'I understand that you want to see the doctor, but he's not available at this time, however I will make sure that he sees you as soon as is possible'.

Education

Healthcare workers can offer education to patients and families about a variety of topics including anger management. Greater understanding about the causes of violence and aggressive acts may help to prevent such behaviour by clarifying misunderstandings and inviting the patient to consider other alternatives.

Written information and advice

As part of the education process, staff may ask the patient to read a particular pamphlet or article on anger management. The healthcare worker and patient then discuss what was read and decide which, if any, of the ideas the patient might be able to use when angry or aggressive.

Relaxation training

Relaxation is an integral part of many interventions designed to help people deal with feelings of tension and stress, anger and frustration. The most commonly taught methods are based on learning how to contract and relax groups of muscles systematically, coupled with learning how to control breathing. Other methods rely on visualisation of a pleasant place or event, perhaps under the direction of a therapist – a technique known as guided fantasy.

Training in controlled breathing may be particularly helpful for people who suffer from panic attacks. Howard believes that hyperventilation is an important component of panic and contributes to some of the symptoms because it reduces the amount of carbon dioxide in the blood.[43] Slow, controlled breathing is, incompatible with hyperventilation. Patients taught this skill can then learn to use it to moderate their feelings of panic.

Teaching relaxation skills to patients is not difficult, but it does take time and commitment.[43] The use of printed handouts can considerably reduce the contact time between nurse or doctor and patient. Cassette tapes, CDs, videos and DVDs on relaxation can be bought quite cheaply these days and could be kept as a resource to loan out to patients.

Activity 4.2

Reflect on your workplace. How well could a violent incident be managed? Would help readily be available? How easy would it be to retreat from an attack?

Contracting

A contract is a written document that is developed by the healthcare professional and patient. In the document, information is clearly stated about acceptable and unacceptable behaviours, consequences and rewards, and the role of both the patient and nurse in preventing and managing aggressive behaviour.

Limit setting and time out

Limit setting as a therapeutic tool is a non-punitive, non-manipulative act in which the patient is told what behaviour is acceptable, what is not acceptable, and the consequences of behaving unacceptably. Research has shown that it is possible to prevent some of a patient's anger by improving staff limit-setting styles.[44] The healthcare worker does not assume responsibility for the patient's behaviour, adaptive or maladaptive. It is recognised that the patient has the right to choose behaviour and knows the consequences of it. Limits should be clarified before negative consequences are applied.

Once a limit has been identified, the consequences must take place if the behaviour occurs. Every staff member must be aware of the plan and carry it out consistently. If staff do not do so, the patient is likely to manipulate staff by acting out and then pointing out areas of inconsistent limit setting. Clear, firm, and non-punitive enforcement of limits is the goal. It is important to understand that when limit setting is implemented, the maladaptive behaviour will not immediately decrease. In fact, it may briefly increase. This is consistent with behavioural principles and testing behaviour. If staff understand the dynamics of the intervention they will understand that the patient's behaviour will eventually change. In a mental health setting it is essential that the nurse makes behavioural limits and consequences clear. Whenever possible, consequences should be matched to the interests and desires of the patient.

Time out from reinforcement is a behavioural technique in which socially inappropriate behaviours can be decreased by short-term removal of the patient from over-stimulating and sometimes reinforcing situations. Time out is most effective with patients who feel loss of social contact as a negative consequence. With time out, patients have more control over the process, and thus this intervention offers an alternative that involves less humiliation and less risk of injury.

Supervision

This is the continuous assessment and observation of a patient, with a readiness to intervene in the event of deterioration in the person's functioning. Consideration needs to be given over to the type and ratio of carers required to carry out the supervision, based on clinical risk and minimum level of safety compatible with good management. Intervention should follow the principles of de-escalation, with restraint and seclusion as a last resort.

Seclusion

Seclusion is the removal of a patient to a designated room in response to immediate violence or threat of injury, both to self or others. The patient is kept in isolation and the room locked. Seclusion of a patient is rightly covered by legislation, and those providing such care should be trained in its use. The room itself is specially designed for the purpose it serves, which is to provide a safe and secure environment. The use of seclusion has little if any therapeutic value, and should only be used as a last resort for the minimum time required.

Breakaway

Breakaway, like physical restraint, should only be used by those trained in such techniques and always as a last resort. Breakaway is useful for the most common of attacks and incorporates leverage rather than strength, as a means of escape. These techniques enable an individual to disengage a variety of common holds used by a stronger aggressor.

Self-defence training

Although a popular growth industry in the UK, there is little evidence for the efficiency of self-defence training. Like so many activities associated with the management of violence and aggression, there is concern as to the type and nature of the self-defence that is being taught. While an increase in confidence has been reported following such training, the issue remains one of practical use within a care environment, and might cause harm to the assailant or expose the person to more serious injury and attack. Particular concern has been expressed as to the material and learning contained within self-defence training videos/DVDs and books. Many of the techniques taught appear to be extremely violent in nature, and include very little if any information about defusing violent situations, and they should be avoided.

Control and restraint

Restraint has been defined as the deprivation or restriction of liberty, freedom of action, or movement.[45] In broad terms, it means restricting someone's liberty or preventing them from doing something they want to do. In general, restraint is described as an intervention that prevents a person from behaving in 'ways that threaten or cause harm to themselves, others or to property'.[46] This can be executed in many ways, for example, by means of physical force whereby the individual is manually restrained by others (nurses, doctors, etc), or through the use of medication which may affect the individual's ability to mobilise freely.[45] Restraint can also be applied by using apparatus or equipment such as door locks to keep an individual restricted within a particular area,[47] or by more subtle means such as reducing heating or comfortableness in certain rooms within the ward, to discourage use of these areas at specific times.[48]

Research also suggests that decisions on the use or avoidance of restraints are made in response to the behaviour of clients.[14] Behaviours that typically lead to the decision to apply restraint have been described by nursing staff as disruptive, difficult, asocial, bizarre, deviant or inappropriate. A common denominator of all these labels is that the behaviour has been identified through interaction with others.[33] It always appears problematic in the environment concerned, and has negative effects for the patients themselves, other residents or staff. As such, behaviour is relative to the context in which it occurs as well as to the interpreter of the act. This means that the behaviour of clients that might be perfectly normal in the home environment may be defined as disruptive in an institution, depending on who is making the judgement. From this point it might be useful to evaluate the behaviours of individuals as relational, rather than examining them from a personal or disease-related viewpoint.

The use of control and restraint is, and always will be, an emotive issue. Some argue for its complete abolition, while others argue that it is sometimes the only way of ensuring the safety and wellbeing of clients and staff, for example, to prevent serious injury. It is clear that interventions that address patients' clinical needs, and those that seek to reduce the risk of violence by improving quality of life and care are preferable. No one would deny that understanding and addressing patient distress must be central to the caring relationship. However, there may still be times when it is necessary to impose control on a patient's behaviour to prevent or minimise harm. The very act of restraint may have a counter-productive effect by actually escalating violent and aggressive behaviour instead of calming a situation and reducing the risk of harm to both patient and staff.[49]

Every citizen who is not subject to legal detention has the right to be free from the use of unauthorised force to restrict his or her speech or movement. Anyone who is restrained (whatever their mental or physical condition) is being denied a fundamental human right, though there may be circumstances where there are other over-riding considerations.

Anyone who applies any form of restraint should be prepared and able to justify why they have done it. The action is unlikely to be unlawful provided that it can be shown to be the only way of preventing harm to the individual or others, it is used for a short time only, and it is regularly reviewed with the client and, where appropriate, significant others, and the multidisciplinary team.

There are a number of circumstances in which nurses are empowered by law to use restraint. Certain sections of the 1983 Mental Health Act and the 1986 Mental Health (Northern Ireland) Order allow the use of restraint for specific purposes, and nurses have the same rights as other citizens to use the minimum restraint necessary to prevent a crime occurring.

When using restraint, staff should be mindful of the risk of abusing the client. The potential for abusive treatment of patients is obvious, and there are several aspects of physical restraint that are of particular concern. Firstly, there is the issue of pain compliance. Some approaches to physical restraint (perhaps most notably the approaches to control and restraint which are taught and used within the prison service and special hospitals) immobilise the arms by employing joint locks which involve wrist flexation. These allow the administration of pain in order to induce compliance in unco-operative patients who are being restrained in this manner. Some commentators are very critical of this, objecting to the idea that nurses should inflict pain on those that they care for.[50] A related criticism is that the notion of applying controlled pain implies an exact titration that is unlikely to be achieved in practice. Indeed, some patients may have conditions (such as learning disabilities and intoxification) in which pain perception and tolerance may be altered, thereby increasing the risk of excessive pain being experienced (where the pain threshold is low) or of injury (where the pain threshold is high). Even where pain compliance is not used, the threat of pain that is implicit in the use of such locking techniques still makes their use ethically objectionable. However, the use of immobilisation techniques which do not lock the joints is becoming more widespread (for example, modified C&R* systems), although some degree of discomfort may be inevitable by the very nature of attempting to exert physical control of a resistive person. Staff should be aware of this possibility and therefore should attempt to prevent or reduce discomfort as much as possible.

Using physical restraint is not without its risks. The placement of patients in the prone position can clearly be dangerous. Indeed one of the recommendations is that the holding of a patient in the prone position should be avoided or at least imposed for no more than three minutes, as breathing difficulties could result as a consequence of this. Similarly, little attention has been given to the use of medication with physical restraint. This again raises the issue of asphyxiation, particularly when used in tandem with holds that may obstruct the airway, such as in the management of the patient's head.

A further issue is the possibility that some techniques and practices compromise the dignity of patients, or may mirror and replicate previous traumatic experiences (particularly physical or sexual abuse). Beside pain compliance, these include taking the patient to the floor and restraining him/her there, holding the trunk (e.g. 'bear hugs'), techniques which push the patient's face to the floor.[51]

---

* Control and restraint is used to describe a range of techniques employed in order to exercise control over a person who is a risk to themselves or others.

While alternatives to most of these techniques exist, it might not always be possible to use them. For example, while restraining in a chair or seated on a bed is considered more socially acceptable than restraining on the floor,[42] a bed or appropriate seating might not always be readily available, or if it is, it might be necessary to restrain the patient on the ground before it can be reached. Staff should therefore take the opportunity to discuss any issues the incident has brought up for patients who have been restrained (which may include guilt and relief as well as any retraumatisation) and attempt to resolve them, as well as discussing why restraint was necessary and other means of addressing the causes of the incident.

Methods of restraint[46]

- Bedrails/cocoon beds/hammocks
- Inappropriate bed height (too high or too low)
- Harnesses
- Medication
- Baffle locks
- Locked doors
- Inappropriate use of wheelchair safety straps
- Arranging furniture to impede movement
- Using bean bags for seating
- Stair gates
- Inappropriate use of night clothes during waking hours
- Chairs whose construction immobilises clients, including reclining chairs
- Isolation
- Controlling language, body language and non-verbal behaviour
- Removal of outdoor shoes and other walking aids
- Withdrawal of sensory aids such as spectacles
- Electronic tagging

Mechanical restraint

The use of mechanical restraints has largely been discredited in the UK and is considered bad practice in all but the most extreme of circumstances where a patient has been judged to be a danger to self and others and where other methods of calming the patient have failed. Recently a government interdepartmental group charged with addressing the needs of violent patients and inmates held talks with an American company Handle With Care which sells a range of restraining products including the 'ParaBed' that secures a patient's arms, feet and torso, leaving them incapable of movement.[52] While such restraint is not advocated here, it has caused a degree of debate, which is set to rise, amongst health professionals and client interest groups as to how best to serve those individuals who use extreme violence as a means of expression.

Pin-down

This is an outdated form of physical restraint first developed for use with disturbed children. It looked to control the child by controlling all four limbs, which were held fast until they became calm and by turn compliant. Rather than being used as a means of promoting safety it developed to include a range of sanctions and was at times used as punishment, so much so in fact, that current guidance prohibits this technique.

Rapid tranquillisation

Violence by patients presents a serious risk both to themselves and to others. Quick safe and effective pharmacological intervention is often required. Rapid tranquillisation is defined as the procedure for giving various amounts of antipsychotic medication over brief intervals of time to control agitated, threatening and potentially destructive patients. The National Institute for Health and Clinical Excellence published guidelines on the use of rapid tranquillisation and management of imminent violence.[53,54] As part of these reports the evidence on effective rapid tranquillisation was systematically reviewed.

Rapid tranquillisation, physical intervention and seclusion should only be considered once de-escalation and other strategies have failed to calm the service user. These interventions are management strategies and are not regarded as primary treatment techniques. When determining which interventions to employ, clinical need, safety of service users and others, and, where possible, advance directives should be taken into account. The intervention selected must be a reasonable and proportionate response to the risk posed by the service user.

Finally, locked units, inflexible unit structures, and non-therapeutic milieus can increase the risk for assaultive behaviour, by suggesting that aggressive behaviour is acceptable or even expected. Overly strict unit structure may render staff unable to respond to patients empathically. In turn, patients may perceive the unit as coercive, controlling, and threatening, and feel that behavioural options are limited to disruptive, desperate, or violent acts. Such settings often provoke the very behaviour they are intended to control.

Treatment outcomes can be considered at both individual and aggregated levels. The desired outcome at the individual level is that the patient is able to gain or maintain control over their aggressive thoughts, feelings and actions. The nurse may observe that the patient shows decreased psychomotor activity (e.g. less pacing of the floor), has a more relaxed posture, speaks more directly about feelings of anger and personal needs, requires less sedating medication, shows increase tolerance for frustration and the ability to consider alternatives, and makes effective use of other coping strategies.

Evidence of a reduction of risk factors may include decreased noise and confusion in the immediate environment, calmness on the part of nursing staff and others, and a climate of clear expectations and mutual acceptance and respect. In unit, day hospital, or group home settings, indicators of positive treatment outcomes might be a reduction in the number of assaults on staff and other patients, a decrease in the number of incident reports, and increased staff competency in de-escalating potentially violent situations.

References

1 Pollock N, McBain I and Webster CD. Clinical decision making and the assessment of dangerousness. In: Howells K and Hollins CR (eds). *Clinical Approaches to Violence*. Chichester: John Wiley; 1989.

2 Wykes T (ed). *Violence and Health Care Professionals*. London: Chapman and Hall; 1994.

3 Whittington R. Violence to nurses: prevalence and risk factors. *Nursing Standard*. 1997; **12**: 49–56.

4 Leather P, Brady C, Lawrence C *et al.* (eds). *Work-related Violence. Assessment and intervention*. London: Routledge; 1999.

5 Ohon N. Workplace violence: theories of causation and prevention strategies. *Journal of the American Association of Occupational Health Nurses*. 1994; **4**: 477–82.

6 Delaney J, Cleary M, Jordan R *et al.* An exploratory investigation into nursing management of aggression in acute psychiatric settings. *Journal of Psychiatric and Mental Health Nursing*. 2001; **8**: 77–84.

7 Bibby P. *Personal Safety for Health Care Workers*. Aldershot: Arena; 1995.

8 Morrison E. A hierarchy of aggressive and violent behaviours among psychiatric inpatients. *Hospital and Community Psychiatry*. 1992; **43**: 505.

9 National Institute of Occupational Safety and Health (NIOSH). NIOSH Current Intelligence Bulletin 57. *Violence in the Workplace: risk factors and prevenetion strategies*; London: National Institute of Occupational Safety and Health; 1996.

10 Royal College of Nursing. *Dealing with Violence against Nursing Staff: an RCN guide for nurses and managers*. London: Royal College of Nursing; 2002.

11 Occupational Safety and Health Administration. *Guidelines for Preventing Workplace Violence for Health and Social Service Workers*. Washington, DC: Occupational Safety and Health Administration; 1998.

12 Turnbull J and Paterson B. *Aggression and Violence: approaches to effective management*. London: MacMillan; 1999.

13 Hamolia CC. Preventing and managing aggressive behaviour. In: Stuart GW and Laraia MT. *Principles and Practice of Psychiatric Nursing* (6e) London: Mosby; 2004.

14 Janelli LM. Physical restraint use in acute care settings. *Journal of Nursing Care Quality*. 1995; **9**: 86–92.

15 Kaplan SG and Wheeler EG. Survival skills for working with potentially violent client. *Social Casework*. 1983; **64**: 339–45.

16 Royal College of Psychiatrists. *Safety for Trainees in Psychiatry*. Council report CR78. London: Royal College of Psychiatrists; 1999.

17 Cowin L, Davies R, Estall G *et al.* De-escalating aggression and violence in the mental health setting. *International Journal of Mental Health Nursing*. 2003; **12**: 64–73.

18 Stirling C. Natural therapeutic holding: a non-aversive alternative to the use of control and restraint in the management of violence for people with learning disabilities. *Journal of Advanced Nursing*. 1997; **26**: 304–11.

19 Cembrowicz S, Ritter S and Wright S. *Violence in Healthcare: understanding, preventing and surviving violence: a practical guide for health professionals* (2e). Oxford: Oxford University Press; 2001.

20 Bulatao E, Q Vanden, Bos GR. Workplace violence: its scope and the issues. In: Vanden Bos GR and Bulatao EQ (eds). *Violence on the Job*. Washington, DC: American Psychological Association; 1996.

21 Health Service Advisory Committee. *Violence and Aggression to Staff in Health Services*. Guidance on assessment and management. London, HSE Books; 1997.

22 Farrell GA. Therapeutic response to verbal abuse. *Nursing Standard*. 1992; **6**: 29–31.

23 Ellis R, Gates R and Kenworthy N. *Interpersonal Communication in Nursing*. London: Churchill Livingstone; 1995.

24 Garnham P. Understanding and dealing with anger, aggression and violence. *Nursing Standard*. 2001; **16**: 37–42.

25 Di Martino V, Hoel H and Cooper CL. *Preventing Violence and Harassment in the Workplace*. Dublin: European Foundation for the Improvement of Living and Working Conditions; 2003.

26 Stuart GW and Laraia MT. *Principles and Practice of Psychiatric Nursing* (6e). New York: Mosby; 1998.

27 Boyd MA and Nihart MA. *Psychiatric Nursing: contemporary practice* (5e). Philadelphia: Lippicott; 1998.

28 Lanza ML. *Violence against nurses in hospital*. In: Vaden Bos GR and Butatato EQ (eds). *Violence On The Job: identifying risks and developing solutions*. Washington DC: American Psychological Association; 1996.

29 Rich A and Parker D. Reflection and critical incident analysis: ethical and moral implications of their use within nursing and midwifery education. *Journal of Advanced Nursing*. 1995; **22**: 1050–7.

30 Leadbetter D and Paterson P. De-escalating aggressive behaviour. In: Kidd B and Stark C (eds). *Management of Violence and Aggression in Health Care*. London: Gaskell Press; 1995.

31 Argyle M. *Bodily Communication*. London: Methuen; 1988.

32 Olsen DP. When the patient causes the problem: the effect of patient responsibility on the nurse-patient relationship. *Journal of Advanced Nursing*. 1997; **26**: 515–22.

33 Hantikainen V. Nursing staff perceptions of the behaviour of older nursing home residents and decision making on restraint use: a qualitative and interpretative study. *Journal of Clinical Nursing*. 2001; **10**: 246–256.

34 United Kingdom Central Council for Nursing, Midwifery and Health Visiting. *The Recognition, Prevention and Therapeutic Management of Violence*. London: United Kingdom Central Council for Nursing, Midwifery and Health; 2001.

35 Morrall P. Social factors affecting communication. In: Ellis R, Gates R and Kenworthy N. *Interpersonal Communication in Nursing*. London: Churchill Livingstone; 1995.

36 Hindle SA. Psychological factors affecting communication. In: Ellis R, Gates R and Kenworthy N. *Interpersonal Communication in Nursing*. London: Churchill Livingstone; 1995.

37 Crawford P and Brown B. Communication. In: Mallik M, Hall C and Howard D. (eds). *Nursing Knowledge and Practice: foundations for decision making* (2e). London: Baillière Tindall; 2004.

38 Goffman I. *The Presentation of Self in Everyday Life*. London: Penguin; 1969.

39 Watkins P. *Mental Health Nursing: the art of compassionate care*. Oxford: Butterworth Heinemann; 2001.

40 McKay J, Daws M and Fanning P. *Messages (Communication Skills)*. London: New Harbinger Publications; 1983.

41 Farrell GA and Gray C. *Aggression: a nurse's guide to therapeutic management*. London: Scutari Press; 1992.

42 McDonnell A, McEvoy J and Dearden RL. Coping with violent situations in the caring environment. In: Wykes T (ed). *Violence and Health Care Professionals*. London: Chapman and Hall; 1994.

43 Howard D. Stress, relaxation and rest. In: Mallik M, Hall C and Howard D (eds). *Nursing Knowledge and Practice: foundations for decision making* (2e). London: Baillière Tindall; 2004.

44 National Institute for Mental Health. *Mental Health Policy Implementation Guide: developing positive practice to support the safe and therapeutic management of aggression*. London: National Institute for Mental Health; 2002.

45 Brennen S. Dangerous liaisons. *Nursing Times*. 1999; **95**: 30–2.

46 Royal College of Nursing. *Restraint Revisited – Rights, Risk and Responsibility: guidance for nursing staff.* London: Royal College of Nursing; 2004.

47 Horsburgh D. The ethical implications and legal aspects of patient restraint. *Nursing Times.* 2003; **99**: 29–34.

48 Tarbuck P. Use and abuse of control and restraint. *Nursing Standard.* 1992; **6**: 30–2.

49 Stirling C and McHugh A. Natural therapeutic holding: a non-aversive alternative to the use of control and restraint in the management of violence for people with learning disabilities. *Journal of Advanced Nursing.* 1997; **26**: 304–11.

50 Shinbach SK and Hayes P. Are we too quick to use restraints? *Registered Nurse.* 1986; **49**: 18–20.

51 Paterson B, Leadbetter D and McCormish A. De-escalation in the management of aggression and violence. *Nursing Times.* 1997; **93**: 58–61.

52 O'Hara M. Straitjacket may be brought back into NHS. *The Guardian*: February 2; 2005.

53 National Institute for Health and Clinical Excellence (NICE). *Violence-rapid Tranquillisation.* London: National Institute for Health and Clinical Excellence; 2004.

54 National Institute for Health and Clinical Excellence (NICE) *The Short-term Management of Disturbed/Violent Behaviour in In-patient Psychiatric Settings and Emergency Departments.* London: National Institute for Health and Clinical Excellence; 2005.

Chapter 5

Staff support

Post-incident support

Responding to staff after an incident should not be seen as a separate issue but part of the overall policy in preventing and controlling violence and aggression at work.[1] This includes the immediate response action needed to manage the consequences of an act of aggression and also the follow-up and evaluation of what happened so that lessons can be learnt for the future. An effective, sensitive response is crucial if people are to cope with the longer-term impact of such acts and adjust to everyday life once again.[2]

Ways of coping

People develop different ways of coping during the course of their life.[3] They learn to manage the demands made of them and exercise control over their choice and decision making. Lifestyles are built around patterns of response that have been established to cope with stressful situations and threats.[4] These lifestyles are highly individual and necessary to protect and maintain a person's sense of wellbeing.

When challenged, people will often revert to coping strategies that have proved successful over time and from which they have found reward.[5] Coping activities take a wide variety of forms including all diverse behaviours that people engage in to meet actual or anticipated challenges. Available coping mechanisms are those that people usually use when they have a problem. They may sit down and try to think the problem through or talk it over with a friend. Some might cry out their frustrations or try to get rid of their feelings of anger and hostility by swearing, kicking a chair, or slamming a door. Others may get into verbal battles with family and friends. Some may react by temporarily withdrawing from the situation in order to reassess the problem, while others will throw themselves into some form of activity in an effort not to think about their problem or difficulty. These are just a few of the many coping methods people use to relieve tension and anxiety when faced with a problem. Each has been used at some time in the developmental past of the individual, has been found effective in maintaining emotional control and has become part of his or her lifestyle in meeting and dealing with the stresses of daily living.[5]

Responding to violence and aggression

The initial response to aggression is a physiological one, with high levels of arousal and emotional upset. The person may be responding to external demands, such as keeping control of the situation, and it may be some hours before the actual impact of the event is apparent. This initial set of reactions can include psychological shock, numbness, confusion, and disorientation, heightened feelings of fear, vulnerability, helplessness, dependency and anger. It is not unusual for staff to blame themselves for the assault or to question their competence in managing potentially violent patients. Often people will ask 'Could I have done things differently?' or 'Was I to blame for the incidence?' In the long term, the staff member might experience sleep loss, appetite change and related fatigue, as well as, flashbacks and intrusive memories of the event. There might be a loss of vocation and the person may go off sick or leave the service altogether.

These feelings and thoughts are normal responses to abnormal circumstances and are generally short-lived. However, there is always the possibility that such feelings and thoughts could develop into something more disabling as in post-traumatic stress disorder or psychological burnout. It is assumed that the greater the frequency and the graver the form of violence, the more severe the reaction to it. This need not be the case, as individuals will vary in their perception of the event and their ability to cope with the situation.

It is important therefore that having been involved in an incident, individuals are allowed to recover and receive help and support. Healthcare workers can be supported by being allowed adequate time off from work to address their physical and emotional needs. Discussing the event in a non-blaming manner can also be helpful. Validation from others that assaults occur despite clinical competence and appropriate interventions can help staff in the healing process. The important thing is that having been involved in a violent or aggressive incident, individuals are allowed to recover and receive practical help and support. Even after minor incidents, feelings may be difficult to control and may affect the ability to deal with further problems. Whatever support is offered should provide a means by which the staff member can work through their feelings and start to make sense of what happened to them.

Following an attack

Following any kind of attack there is a need to introduce a cooling off period when things are allowed to return back to normal. This enables a sense of control and stability to emerge and is the first step in the recovery process. Assistance should be given to helping the person complete the necessary documentation as well as providing practical help and support. This might mean the administration of first aid as well as picking up the person's work duties or caseload.

It is important to remember that violent incidents in the workplace can also have an impact on those that observed it. Witnessing violence may lead to fear of future violent incidents and as such has similar negative effects as being personally assaulted or attacked.[6] Opportunity should therefore be given to explore the incident either formally and/or informally. The most practical approach to this, and one often pursued in practice, is to gather those staff who were involved to talk about what happened, allowing them to explore what they feel about the incident and the way in which it was managed.

Cembrowicz and Ritter suggest that three meetings should take place:[7]

1   an informal meeting as soon after the event as possible to discuss what happened and how people are feeling
2   a meeting (no more than 1–2 days after the event) to discuss formally what happened and how people are feeling
3   a meeting to address both issues arising from the last meeting and also future action plans/ways of working.

Healthcare workers are not usually good at identifying and meeting their own needs,[8,9] wanting to 'just get on with the job', and there might be a reluctance to engage in initiatives of this kind following an aggressive episode, however participation should be encouraged. Group discussions, such as those listed above, can be particularly effective as a means of sharing experience, concerns and feelings. They can help to ensure that staff do not feel isolated and are aware that there are others with similar reactions and fears.

Debriefing

A debrief should be considered for all those involved in an aggressive or violent incident. This should be to establish the facts as to what had happened and to allow time for staff to talk through their feelings on the matter. The debriefing process involves groups of people witnessing an incident recounting their impressions and understanding of the event in a systematic and structured form. It is designed to enable the person to re-experience the incident in a controlled and safe environment in order to make sense of and become reconciled with the traumatic event. It has been shown that debriefing can prevent the development of adverse reactions to trauma by giving back the perception of control over their life.[10] The control is achieved by enabling the victim to integrate, at a cognitive level, the profound personal experiences brought about by the trauma.[11] In situations where there are a number of people involved in an incident, the sharing of feelings and information in a group debrief is particularly useful as it enables the individuals involved to feel less isolated, reduces the likelihood of scapegoating, and encourages acceptance of reactions to the trauma as natural.[12] The opportunity for catharsis through the disclosure of traumatic events is suggested to lead to a reduction in arousal and improved immune functioning.[12] Cembrowicz and Ritter stress the importance of the debrief as a way of allowing the person to gain mastery over their emotions by actively redefining the experience and its consequences, this mastery enabling the individual to distance themselves from the event, allowing the traumatic experience to be brought to a conclusion.[7]

How a debriefing is conducted and the form that it takes will be very much down to the individuals involved and the resources available to them. At a minimum level all staff should be provided with the opportunity to vent their emotions and thoughts on the matter and to be reassured that support will be available to them in the future if they need it. Conducting a debriefing requires skills and knowledge, and should be led by someone competent in such matters. Disclosure of the kind described within an aggressive incident can be a painful experience for the individual involved, bringing things to consciousness that need dealing with. The memory of a challenging situation often includes an affective component, so people involved in the debrief should be aware of and comfortable with the affective responses of others. Some incidents may be so challenging that they create a great deal of uncontrolled emotion, and cathartic support may be necessary before an attempt to think positively or constructively becomes possible. Another important point is to know when to refer on. If someone has been either physically or psychologically damaged then psychological support from skilled professionals may need to be arranged.

The Institute of Counselling suggests that:[13]

- debriefing should be done by a person with the necessary experience in stress management
- only people with direct experience of the incident should be present
- debriefing is not the evaluation of the behaviour but a time for sharing thoughts, feelings and experiences
- people are warned that they may feel worse at first talking about the experience
- those who provide support to people following a critical incident need recognition, support, stress relief, supervision and time to record their experience when the time is right
- individual counselling may need to be offered to help people to work through their personal experiences
- debriefing is not seen as counselling.

Reviewing the incident

The purpose of a review is to take positive learning from the incident to reduce the likelihood of a similar situation happening again, and to see how such incidents could be managed more effectively, if at all. Littlechild suggests that strategies for managing aggression should exist at three levels: with practitioners, with managers and at an agency level.[14] This structure should form the basis of a review:

- at *practitioner level* opportunities are present for individuals to learn from their experience and they need to adopt different and modified personal strategies
- at *manager level* learning points can be identified and questions concerning issues such as the availability and skill of help provided and the speed of response should be asked
- at *agency level* issues of policy amendment or change may need to be addressed and the effectiveness and availability of post-incident support can be identified.

Acknowledging the healthcare worker's right to take legal action against the patient can also be helpful. In fact, many argue that it is therapeutic to bring criminal charges against assaultive patients. Legal action can help patients take responsibility for their behaviour, and perhaps decrease future violent episodes. For the assaulted staff member, taking legal action articulates a position that the personal trauma of being physically assaulted should not be an accepted consequence of caring for others.

From the above it appears that following a critical incident these points need to be taken into consideration:

- debriefing of some kind needs to be offered
- it needs to be facilitated by someone who has the necessary experience
- blame is not the aim, but an action plan to prevent it happening again can provide some resolution for those involved
- expression of thoughts, feelings, perceptions and effects on the normal activity of living needs to be encouraged
- individual help needs to be made available for those who need it
- those involved in facilitating the debrief also need support and supervision
- all of the above is dependent on external factors including, managerial responsibility, availability of staff, willingness to work towards a team approach and current relationships within the team.

Staff must also receive continued support when they return to work after a violent incident. Individuals may feel the impact of workplace violence and aggression more acutely on site because they are at the place where the violence took place. The person responsible for supervising the staff member must look out for any residual effects that the incident may be having, such as reduced self-confidence and satisfaction with work.

Those affected by the emotional consequences of experiencing violence at work are likely to take these experiences home with them. The kinds of support available through relationships with family and friends vary. Those experiencing strained relationships at home may feel more acute consequences of anxiety and threat at work.

Reflective practice

An adjunct to the debriefing session is the use of reflective practice. Reflective practice allows the member of staff to consciously consider their experiences through the integration of theory with practice and in turn, with praxis, through experience. Reflection involves defining a problem, asking questions, examining evidence, analysing assumptions and biases, confronting emotional unease, considering other interpretations, and tolerating ambiguity. It requires constructing new knowledge and new ways of thinking by perceiving a dilemma, exploring the differing perspectives, integrating existing knowledge and considering new alternatives. Reflection can be undertaken on an individual basis or through clinical supervision.

The following model offers a series of questions to help the staff member reflect on their experience:[15]

Phenomenon

- Describe the event in the sequence that it happened.

Causal

- What caused the event to happen as it did?

Context

- What were the significant background factors to this experience?

Reflection

- What was I trying to achieve?
- Why did I intervene as I did?
- What were the consequences of my actions for:
  - myself?
  - the patient/family?
  - the people that I work with?
- How did I feel about the experience when it was happening?
- How did the patient feel about it?
- How do I know how the patient felt about it?
- What factors/knowledge influenced my decisions and actions?

Alternative actions

- What other choices did I have?
- What would be the consequences of these other choices?

Learning

- How do I feel now about the experience?
- Could I have dealt better with the experience?
- What have I learned from the experience?

Clinical supervision

Clinical supervision is a broad concept, having been adopted and integrated into many helping professions and has been defined as:

> A formal process of professional support and learning which enables individual practitioners to develop knowledge and competence, assume responsibility for their own practice and enhance consumer protection and safety of care in complex clinical situations. It is central to the process of learning and to the scope of the expansion of practice and should be seen as a means of encouraging self-assessment and analytical and reflective skills.[16]

Clinical supervision brings practitioners and skilled supervisors together to reflect on practice. The supervisor is primarily there to ensure that the client gets the best possible care by helping the member of staff to identify solutions to problems, improve practice, and increase understanding of professional issues. Indicators of benefit could include safer practice; reduced untoward incidents and complaints; improved confidence and self-worth.

Internal supervision

Casement suggests that professionals develop their own supervision within themselves, called the internal supervisor.[17] Developing an ability to process helping interventions at the same time as engaging in them is a requirement of the effective healthcare worker. Self-awareness of this kind enables a person to analyse their own feelings, beliefs and values through everyday work situations. Dexter and Wash state that being honest with yourself about your self-doubt and personal limitations can help reduce 'personal pressures' of having to do something well.[18]

Stress and psychological burnout

Violence and aggression can cause stress and psychological burnout. It is important to understand and recognise the psychological and mental harm that this can cause to the person, and the care and support that they deliver. There is the perception that healthcare workers should be able to cope with the most adverse of circumstances and not be affected by them when they happen, and this is one reason why many incidents of violence and aggression go unreported. Examples of the effects of stress are shown in Table 5.1.[19]

Karasek has suggested a 'demand-discretion' model of occupational stress, whereby the effects of job demands are moderated by job control or discretion.[20] He predicts in his model that:

- a combination of high job demand and low levels of job discretion would lead to high levels of psychological and physical strain
- low job demands and high levels of discretion makes for jobs that are not too stressful, allowing the person to develop protective barriers
- jobs with low demands and low discretion tend to be passive and result in reduced activity and learned helplessness.

This approach suggests, therefore that people need to have a sense of control over their work, balanced by reasonable demands. Too many/not enough demands, and little control can cause stress.

Warr identified a number of environmental features that could affect a person's mental health and wellbeing.[21] They are:

- *opportunity for control*: how much control a person has over their time and incidents that occur
- *opportunity for skill use*: culture for the use of existing skills and the development of new ones
- *externally generated goals*: the level of demands placed on a person in the work environment
- *variety*: the extent of variety in the working environment
- *environmental clarity*: feedback about a person's performance, predictability of the environment, role requirements
- *opportunities for interpersonal contact*: friendship and social support
- *physical security*: job satisfaction and adequate working conditions
- *valued social position*: a person's value as seen and appreciated by peers.

Table 5.1 Examples of the effects of stress[19]

Physical	Mental	Emotional	Behavioural
Headache	Forgetfulness	Discontent	Resisting change/ inflexibility
Indigestion	Poor concentration	Anxiety/worry	Cynicism
Tense, tight muscles, back ache, neck ache	Difficulties with decision making and thinking things through	Apprehensive a lot of the time	Absenteeism
Sleeplessness	Putting oneself down	Tearful	Talking a lot
Menstrual problems	Beating oneself up	Hopelessness	Overworking
Diarrhoea	Imagining the worst	Irritable, annoyed	Losing interest easily
Tiredness, exhaustion	Changing one's mind	Angry more of the time	Apathy, inertia
Restlessness	Feeling confused, muddled	Easily exasperated	Withdrawn
Cold hands and feet	Dreaming a lot	More despondent, sad, depressed	Destructiveness
Trembling		Helplessness	Drinking a lot
Jumpiness		Resentment	Insensitive, impatient with others
Frequency		High, excitable	Avoiding people
Sweating		Doubt/uncertainty	Taking less care with appearance, diet, hygiene
Palpitations			Making mistakes
Tight breathing			Reduced commitment to work
Pallor			Complaining a lot Taking work home 'Busy' syndrome 'Indispensable' syndrome

Table 5.2 Mental defence mechanisms[22]

Mechanism	Definition	Example
Denial	When reality is too unpleasant or painful to face then individuals may deny that it really exists	A woman might deny having been sexually abused within a relationship in order to protect the partner
Displacement	Transferring feelings or actions from their original target to another object that arouses less anxiety	You may have been given a hard time by your boss to whom you are unable to retaliate. When you return home you immediately have a blazing argument with your partner
Intellectualisation	Masking anxiety-arousing feelings by discussing them in a detached, intellectual manner	For people working in life-and-death situations, such as in high-dependency units, this defence mechanism may be necessary for survival. If the emotional bluntness extends into other areas of the individual's lives, however, then the mechanism becomes problematic, for example responding to the emotional needs of a colleague who has been attacked
Projection	Blaming someone else for how you feel	The ward manager who is unable to manage the ward effectively may blame the situation on incompetent staff
Rationalisation	Finding an acceptable explanation for an act that you find unacceptable	'It's in the overall best interest for the patient'; 'You have to be cruel to be kind'
Reaction formation	Concealing what you really feel by thinking and acting in the opposite way.	Some people who have an issue in their life about which they feel uncomfortable may campaign against the issue. For example, individuals who have led promiscuous lives may campaign strongly for the sanctity of family values
Regression	Individuals engaging in behaviours from an earlier, more secure life stage	Losing your temper and engaging in tantrums when things go wrong
Repression	Unconscious exclusion of memories, feelings etc from awareness in order to prevent anxiety or guilt	A person having been attacked may repress the memory of the events leading up to the incident
Sublimation	Redirecting the energy from unacceptable sexual or aggressive drives into another socially acceptable activity	An ambitious member of staff may utilise sublimation to secure promotions at the expense of family and social commitments

In response to stress an individual may attempt to cope by adopting mental defence mechanisms. Defence mechanisms are unconscious processes used to cope with negative emotions as found in sustained aggression such as harassment. In the short term they are a healthy response and they help the individual to survive the immediate period following exposure to the stress. The major defence mechanisms are outlined in Table 5.2.[22]

Defence mechanisms do not alter the cause of the stress, however; they only alter an individual's interpretation of it. They create an illusion and consequently involve a degree of self-deception. The prolonged use of mental defence mechanisms is therefore unhealthy and can interfere in the person's ability to manage further stress such as that brought on by violence and aggression.

Watkins suggests the following ways of managing stress:[19]

- develop problem-solving skills: confront the issue rather than denying, ignoring it or muddling through
- develop assertiveness skills; are your needs being ignored? Are you always saying 'yes' (a problem with carers)?
- be aware of how your thinking about stressful situations adds to your discomfort
- learn and use relaxation skills when in stressful situations
- nurture yourself physically, emotionally, socially, spiritually
- have plenty of distracters and outside interests
- talk things through with others
- develop and maintain a good support system.

Burnout

Burnout occurs because of continued stress. People suffering from burnout often feel that it is because of a weakness on their part. This can be reinforced by attitudes of work colleagues and others who may be less sympathetic. Employers can also reinforce this further by blaming the person rather than addressing the issues that may be causing the stress.[23] Burnout can build up slowly over time unnoticed. The danger here is that the person becomes unmotivated and unable to respond to changes in others and the organisation for which they work, placing themselves and others at risk.

Symptoms of burnout

Maslach and Jackson suggested a burnout model described in three dimensions:[24]

- *emotional exhaustion*: people feel they are emotionally drained and unable to give more energy to their clients
- *reduced personal accomplishment*: people feel unable to deal with problems positively, and play down any achievements
- *depersonalisation*: people feel more isolated and hardened towards others.

As with stress, it is useful to monitor for signs of burnout, and take corrective measures to address such. Welch *et al.* suggest two types of burnout:[25]

1 *short-term*: people may have physical effects and feel run down. This may be relieved by a break from work, such as a holiday or a change in the job they are doing, for example secondment to another department or ward. This type of burnout is reversible and short-lived
2 *long-term*: people suffering from prolonged physical, social and psychological burnout decrease in their cognitive functioning, and a gradual withdrawal from social contact. This can affect both their personal and work life, and the recovery period is long and difficult.

The effects of stress and, in turn, emotional burnout can be potentially harmful, and for this reason it is important that steps are taken to protect staff from violence and aggression. Staff who are finding it difficult to cope with the demands made of them from their work require and deserve the support of their colleagues and those that manage them.

Staff support: development and education

Staff education is important not only in the management of violence and aggression but also as a means of prevention. Raising staff knowledge and awareness ensures that the issue is dealt with in an appropriate and caring manner. Education and training should be offered to all groups of employees and not just those considered being at high risk. In an ever-changing professional environment, appropriate support, supervision and education are essential.

The most common employer action for reducing violence against healthcare workers is training on how to minimise and manage violence. However, inconsistencies across the NHS in the availability of training for staff in preventing and managing violence have been identified, and there is lack of information as to how effective these programmes are for preventing violence.[26]

Related to the anxiety about the frequency of violence and aggression is the discomfort felt by staff at the lack of education and training in this area. Criticism has focused on the need for increased preventative measures and the inadequacy of staff training in the prevention, management and review of aggression and violence.[10]

There have also been questions raised as to the appropriateness of some of the techniques taught, and the method by which these have been delivered.[27] The provision of training is often a key part of an organisation's strategy for tackling workplace violence. However, there is little evidence to indicate which techniques are most effective for preventing and managing violence and the types of control and restraint/physical interventions used. Very few organisations collect data on the effectiveness and relevance of their training programmes. Few can demonstrate the safety or relevance of any non-physical and physical skills taught to staff. Turnbull and Paterson propose that staff training which focuses solely on restraint is unsatisfactory, and examine the collective importance of training in the skills of negotiation and collaboration combined with skills of communication towards the development of therapeutic relationships with service users.[28] Training needs should be monitored and reviewed regularly, and educational courses evaluated for their effectiveness.

Risk reduction requires consideration of educational, environmental, and other factors linked to the development and the implementation of locally agreed and workplace-specific policies and protocols. As a minimum, employers should provide training and education for their staff, and this should be commensurate with the degree of risk they face. This may range from the provision of education/ training for staff in low-risk areas such as operating theatres, medium-risk areas such as accident and emergency, to provision in high-risk areas such as secure units. Policies on education for all staff should address how educational programmes on violence and aggression will be developed and implemented. The issue of orientation and continuing education must be included. Access to these programmes and considering the nature of hours worked by healthcare staff should also be addressed.

There has been some acceptance that strategies to protect staff will need to include training in physical skills for those working in high-risk areas. Such training should address: defusing threatening situations, self-protection, application of restraints without injury to anyone, structure and responsibilities of team members, when and how to seek assistance, staff and patients' rights, and reporting mechanisms.

How employers identify, select, and provide training appropriate to the particular needs of their service has often been an issue of concern, largely due to the way in which this type of training has evolved within the care sector. A major focus for present physical skills training has centred on accident and emergency departments, psychiatric units and disability services. However, course content varies across programmes and there is little information to assist healthcare providers in choosing one programme over another. The lack of an identified structure has meant that people seeking to provide training for their staff have often been left to make informal enquires within their personal networks and contacts. In some cases, this system of personal recommendation has perpetuated inappropriate and outdated training.

Whatever training or educational package is pursued, it should be fit for purpose, that is it should reflect local need, both of staff and service user. It should be clear and transparent in its purpose and communicated to all. It should contain learning outcomes so participants are clear as to what is to be achieved and its content should be as up to date with current thinking as is possible and appropriate. In addition to this, its content should be supported by evidence wherever possible; delivered by creditable staff committed to a model of care based on respect for the individual and other key principle. Above all it should be responsive to feedback and allow for the concerns of staff to be played out.

Training and education can bring about:

- a reduction in the number and type of incidents
- a reduction in the seriousness of incidents
- a reduction in the psychological effects of incidents
- an improved response to incidents
- an improvement in staff morale.

Good training programmes typically cover:[29]

- *theory*: understanding aggression and violence in the workplace
- *prevention*: assessing danger and taking precautions
- *interaction with aggressive people*: in particular, how to get out of danger
- *post-incident action*: reporting, investigation, counselling and follow-up.

Promoting clinical effectiveness

In promoting clinical effectiveness training programmes should:

- encourage the continual development and effective utilisation of a team's knowledge, skills and abilities
- contribute to the promotion of a 'no-blame' culture, where self-reflection and modifying behaviour are encouraged
- build effective relationships through the creation of opportunities for inter-organisation communication and consensus
- promote the sharing of learning and good practice between organisations
- collect, analyse, report and share information to support the planning process
- actively involve patients, listening to what they want and promoting their views.

Employers have a duty to ensure that all their staff are prepared appropriately for their roles (including those working on a part-time basis). Quality service provision depends upon an adequately trained workforce.

Developments in staff training

After a survey by the National Audit Office in 2003, a number of recommendations were made that saw new powers being given to the Counter Fraud and Security Management Service (CFSMS). This body now has operational and policy responsibility for violence and security in the NHS, including leading work on reducing violence and aggression against NHS staff. Prior to this, responsibility had been with the NHS Human Resources Directorate who led on all staff welfare and safety issues under the Improving Working Lives Initiative. As part of this reconfiguration of service a new strategy aimed at reducing violence and aggression within the NHS was launched. This included a training programme on conflict resolution for all NHS staff, and a new national reporting system to record incidents of physical assault as well as a new Legal Protection Unit to increase the prosecution rate.

Quickly following its instigation, the CFSMS launched a national one-day training programme, the National Syllabus for Conflict Resolution.[30] This course is designed for all frontline NHS staff and professionals whose work brings them into contact with members of the public.

At the end of the course delegates are expected to be able to:[30]

- describe common causes of conflict
- describe two forms of 'communication'
- give two examples of how communication can breakdown
- explain three examples of 'communication models' that can assist in conflict resolution
- describe patterns of behaviour they may encounter during different interactions
- give examples of the different warning and danger signs
- give examples of impact factors
- describe the use of distance when dealing with 'conflict'

- explain the use of 'reasonable force' as it applies to conflict resolution (*see* Chapter 8)
- describe different methods of dealing with possible conflict situations.

The syllabus was developed in association with The British Medical Association and The Royal College of Nursing and commenced on 1 April 2004.

In 2005 the NHS Special Management Service (SMS) took this one step further and introduced a further training syllabus in non-physical intervention techniques. Titled 'Promoting safer and therapeutic services', it is designed to equip staff working in mental health and learning disability settings with the necessary skills required to recognise, prevent and manage potentially violent situations.[31]

The course is split over two days. The first day deals with primary prevention; i.e. engagement and communication. The second day deals with risks, rights and responsibilities. Both the National Institute for Health and Clinical Excellence (NICE) guidelines for managing violence and aggression, and the recommendations from the inquiry into the death of David 'Rocky' Bennett, following an incident which led to him being physically restrained, are reflected in the syllabus.[32,33] The syllabus consists of modules or sessions in:

- recognising violence and understanding its causes
- rasing awareness – from staff and service-user perspectives
- the impact of social/ physical environment
- cultural awareness, diversity and racial equality
- de-escalation and communication
- problem solving and risk assessment
- legal and ethical issues
- the importance of post-incident reviews and learning the lesson.

The syllabus will become the minimum standard of training that staff in mental health and learning disability settings must be trained in. While health bodies will be required to ensure their staff are trained, they will be able to choose the method of delivery – for example, their existing in-house trainers or external providers. Familiarisation seminars will be arranged by the NHS SMS to ensure that the training is delivered consistently. The course was piloted during 2005 and is set to become effective in 2006. The syllabus is not simply attempting to deal with violence when it does happen, but is about trying to prevent it from happening in the first place through ensuring that flash points are never reached, that ongoing learning takes place and that risk is effectively managed through drawing from experience of incidents that have occurred in the past.

Training provision of this kind should be applauded and seen as a step forward in the prevention and management of violence and aggression. Concerns about violence and aggression are valid and must be recognised and addressed. Being aware and able to recognise the potential for danger will help staff be prepared. It also ensures that they react to a situation in a positive and proactive manner.

References

1 National Audit Commission. *A Safer Place to Work: protecting NHS hospital and ambulance staff from violence and aggression*. Report by the Controller and Auditor General HC527 Session 2002–03. London: The Stationery Office; 2003.

2 Wkyes T and Mezey G. Counselling for victims of violence. In: Wkyes T (ed). *Violence and Healthcare Professionals*. London: Chapman and Hall; 1994.

3 Lindsay JJ and Anderson CA. From antecedent conditions to violent actions: a general affective aggression model. *Journal of Personality and Social Psychology*. 2000; **26**: 533–47.

4 Ohon N. Workplace violence: theories of causation and prevention strategies. *The Journal of the American Association of Occupational Health Nurses*. 1994; **4**: 477–82.

5 Aguilera DC. Crisis stabilization. In: Worley NK (ed). *Mental Health Nursing in the Community*. London: Mosby; 1997.

6 Leather P, Lawrence C, Beale D *et al*. Exposure to occupational violence and the buffering effects of intra-organisational support. *Work and Stress*. 1998; **12**: 161–78.

7 Cembrowicz S and Ritter S. Attacks on doctors and nurses. In: Shepherds J (ed). *Violence in Health Care: a practical guide to coping and caring for victims*. Oxford: Oxford University Press; 1994.

8 Davis C. How to Survive in one Piece. *Nursing Times*. 2000; **96**: 29.

9 Thomas B. Management strategies to tackle in mental health nursing. *Mental Health Care*. 1997; **1**: 15–17.

10 National Institute for Mental Health Executive. *Mental Health Policy Implementation Guide: developing positive practice to support the safe therapeutic management of aggression*. London: National Institute for Mental Health Executive; 2002.

11 Cembrowicz S, Ritter S and Wright S. *Violence in Healthcare: understanding, preventing and surviving violence: a practical guide for health professionals* (2e). Oxford: Oxford University Press; 2001.

12 Vittasara E. *Violence in Caring, Risk Factors, Outcomes and Support*. Stockholm: National Institute for Working Life; 2004.

13 Institute of Counselling. *Introduction to Stress Management*. Glasgow: College of Counselling; 1996.

14 Littlechild B. The risk of violence and aggression to social work and social work staff. In: Kemshall H and Pritchard H (eds). *Good Practice in Risk Assessment and Risk Management*. London: Jessica Kingsley; 1996.

15 Johns C. Professional supervision. *Journal of Nursing Management*. 1993; **1**: 9–18.

16 Department of Health. *Vision of the Future*. London: Department of Health; 1993

17 Casement P. *On Learning from the Patient*. Hove: Routledge; 1985.

18 Dexter G and Wash M. *Psychiatric Nursing Skills* (2e) London: Chapman and Hall; 1995.

19 Watkins P. *Mental Health Nursing: the art of compassionate care*. Oxford: Butterworth Heinemann; 2001.

20 Karasek RA. Job demands, job decision latitude and mental strain: implications for job design. *Administrative Science Quarterly*. 1979; **24**: 285–308.

21 Warr PB. Job characteristics and Mental Health. In: Warr PB (ed). *Psychology at Work*. London: Penguin Books; 1987.

22 Howard D. Stress, relaxation and rest. In: Mallick M, Hall C and Howard D (eds). *Nursing Knowledge and Practice: foundations for decision making* (2e). London: Baillière Tindall; 2004.

23 Howard D. Stress and anxiety. In: Mallick M, Hall C and Howard D (eds). *Nursing Knowledge and Practice: foundations for decision making* (2e). London: Baillière Tindall; 2004.

24 Maslach C and Jackson SE. The measurement of experienced burnout. *Journal of Occupational Behaviour*. 1981; **2**: 99–103.

25 Welch ID, Mederios DC and Tate GA. *Beyond Burnout: how to enjoy your job again when you've just about had enough*. London: Prentice Hall; 1982.

26 Gooding L. News. *Mental Health Practice*. 2004; **7**: 6.

27 Allan D. Nice guidance, but timing is off. *Mental Health Practice.* 2005; **8**: 14–15.

28 Turnbull J and Paterson B (eds). *Aggression and Violence: approaches to effective management.* London: MacMillan; 1999.

29 British Institute for Learning Disabilities (BILD). *BILD Code of Practice for Trainers in the Use of Physical Interventions.* London: British Institute for Learning Disabilities; 2001.

30 NHS Security Management Service (NHS SMS). *Conflict resolution: the national syllabus: a one-day course for frontline NHS staff.* London: NHS SMS; 2004.

31 Nyberg-Coles M. Promoting safer and therapeutic services. *Mental Health Practice.* 2005; **8**: 16–17.

32 National Institute for Health and Clinical Excellence (NICE). *Disturbed (violent) Behaviour: the short-term management of disturbed (violent) behaviour in in-patient psychiatric settings.* London: NICE; 2005.

33 Blofeld J (chair). *An Independent Inquiry set up under HSG (94)27 into the death of David 'Rocky' Bennett.* Cambridge, Norfolk, Suffolk and Cambridgeshire Strategic Health Authority; 2004.

Chapter 6

Special considerations: care in the community

Working in the community

Care in the community is increasingly becoming an option for many patients. Staff who work within this setting often provide care in isolation of others making them vulnerable to increased risk of violence and aggression.[1] For instance, they may work in areas with which they are unfamiliar, and in some neighbourhoods that are dangerous. They are often required to enter a person's home without the ability to pre-assess the environment, and to deal with people that they have met for the first time.[2] It is therefore important that community staff fully understand the risks involved in their work and take action to reduce these. Not having the immediate support of colleagues requires additional planning and preparation. Essential to this is the ability to assess each situation as if it were new. Extra thought needs to be given over to the issue of safety and security. Community staff need to know that there is a structure in place to help them if they need assistance and that these procedures are able to react to the extraordinary as well as the ordinary.[2]

In keeping with the rest of the book, it is important that safe systems of work be put into place in order to reduce the likelihood of attack or abuse. All efforts should be made to carry out a through and proper risk assessment prior to any visit. Where this is not possible, extreme caution should be exercised on seeing the person for the first time. If a home visit is not essential for healthcare reasons, seeing the patient as an outpatient may reduce the risk of visiting particular areas or client groups. This simple measure may also help staff decide on the precautions needed in the event of a home visit being made.[3] Where there are known risks, or identified potential risks, about a patient or a location to be visited, every effort should be made to minimise those risks prior to staff visiting. For example, where a home visit cannot be avoided, the appointment should be scheduled for a time of day that affords extra security, such as the morning when parents are around taking their children to school, and when drug activity and drunkenness should be at a minimum. In addition to this, community staff should be prepared to readdress the goals of their visit if the situation is not how they expected it to be, and leave if need be. Staff should not enter any location where they feel threatened or unsafe. However, this is easier said than done, with staff feeling that they have a moral obligation to provide care, regardless of the circumstances.[4] Having made the decision to leave, staff should inform their manager and record the circumstances by which they left. Where there is a known history of violence and aggression or the situation is considered high risk, the community worker should be encouraged to take along a colleague, go by taxi and have the driver wait, or, in some cases, the police. Procedures for evaluating and arranging for such accompaniment must be developed, and training provided as part of good practice and not left until a situation arises.[5]

The use of a 'buddy system'

Use of a 'buddy system' is highly recommended and should at least be considered whenever staff feel insecure regarding the time of an activity, the location of work, the nature of the client's health problem, patient or family history of aggressive or assaultative behaviour, or potential for aggressive acts.[1–3] A 'buddy' is a nominated colleague who is aware of the other's movements, and acts as a point of contact and source of support. As part of this, community healthcare staff should prepare a daily work plan and keep the nominated contact person informed as to their whereabouts throughout the working day. This reporting system should be consistently adhered to by both parties. Follow-up contacts should be made whenever an employee does not report in at the end of the day or at a designated time. Contingency arrangements should be in place for someone else to take over the 'buddy' role in case the nominated person is called away for whatever reason, or if the situation extends past the end of the nominated person's normal working day or shift. It is also useful to set up systems to ensure exchange of information and co-operation between all agencies that might visit patients in their homes. This can reduce the number of visits made to a persons' house as well as providing a source of support, particularly if joint visits between agencies can be arranged. Such activity should be logged and there must be adequate communication if the system is to be successful. The details of the system should be understood by everyone who has to work it, and must be carried out on each occasion in accordance with what has been agreed.

The use of mobile phones

In order to provide some measure of safety and to facilitate the working of a 'buddy system', mobile phones should be provided for official use when staff go out on visits. There use to be the problem of network coverage, however, this seems to have been addressed in all bar the most remote of places. That said, a mobile phone should not be relied upon as the only means of communication.

Staff should always check the signal strength of their mobile phone before entering a location. If there is no signal, the staff member should contact their manager or colleague ahead of the visit, stating their location and the nature of their visit, along with an estimate of the time they think they will need to spend on the visit. More importantly, the staff member should let whoever they alert know what to do in the event of them not contacting back after the visit. In addition to this, emergency contacts should be kept on speed dial, as this will speed up the process of summoning help. 'Code' words or phases should also be agreed and used that will help the staff member convey the nature of the threat to their managers or colleagues so that they can provide the appropriate response, such as informing the police. For example, ringing base and asking for an address that is kept in the, 'red folder'.[6]

It is also important to note that the use of a mobile phone could potentially be a source of risk. To some patients the use of a mobile phone can prove distracting and a source of agitation and annoyance, especially if it were to keep going off during the course of an interview.[2] It can also provide a target for thieves and therefore should be used with sensitivity.

Hand alarms

Consideration should be given over to the use of hand-held alarms and noise devices. Staff should be trained to use such devices safely and appropriately. Remember such devices are an aid to promoting safety and no more, they will not prevent incidents occurring, and their use in the event of attack is limited.[7] There main use is one of distraction to allow a few precious seconds in which to allow the staff member to make good their escape. The assumption when using an alarm is that there will be no certainty of assistance and that using such a device may increase the chance of attack. The best use of an alarm is to sound it then discard it as the assailant's attention is usually drawn to silencing the device before giving pursuit.[2] As with any piece of equipment, time should be given over to its maintenance and operational capability. If an alarm is carried then it should be kept about the person, in easy reach, ready for use and not concealed in a bag.

Visiting by car

When visiting by car, the community worker should ensure that it has sufficient fuel not only for the journey but also to get away if things went wrong. Employees should be encouraged to carry only absolutely required identification and money. They should not leave any valuables in their car and should leave purses at the office or home. CDs or other equipment should be stored out of sight, preferably in the boot of the vehicle. Allowance should be made for travelling time, to avoid rushing and causing an accident. When travelling, doors should be locked and windows wound up. Staff should always park near to the location that they are visiting and should never take short cuts to save time. At night or in poor weather conditions and visibility, staff should park in a well-lit area facing the direction of travel. They should avoid 'advertising' their service, by not displaying 'on call' signs as this might encourage would be thieves to break into the car in search of drugs etc.[8] Likewise, staff should avoid leaving items containing personal details, such as letters with their home address, in the car, certainly not in public view.

It is recommended by the Health and Safety Executive's safe driving programme that staff do not stop for people who may be in distress or requiring help, but instead contact the emergency services as appropriate. The author knows of an incident where a member of staff stopped to help a distressed woman at the side of the road. On stopping the car, the driver was stabbed by a man who dashed out from where he was hiding and robbed him of his belongings. Staff are also advised to reverse onto patient's driveways, again to ensure that they are facing the direction of travel.[8] If staff feel they are being followed then they should pull into the nearest populated building such as a supermarket and request assistance.

Always have car keys in hand when leaving the person's home, this saves time in looking for keys while standing outside the vehicle, thereby reducing the risk to personal safety. Once inside the vehicle, lock all doors especially when travelling at slow speeds and stopping at traffic light controls. If a visit is regular, vary the time and day to avoid becoming a target.

Transporting clients

Sometimes it is necessary to transport clients, for example, from their home to hospital. Consideration must be given to the most appropriate mode of transport to meet the individual's needs. Never escort a person alone, however urgent the need to do so. Other factors include:[6]

- the number of staff needed
- the risk involved in transporting the patient
- male staff must be present if male patients are being escorted and vice versa for female patients
- where escorting by car always sit patients behind the passenger seat (with seat belt on); staff should always sit behind the driver of the vehicle
- if the patient becomes violent or aggressive pull over and leave the vehicle, having removed the keys. Contact the police as soon as possible.

Visiting a person's home

As is good practice, all community staff should take every step to ensure that they arrive on time for their appointment. In support of this, staff should be made aware of policy changes and administrative problems (such as change of appointments) which may upset clients and elicit aggravated responses.[9] Ringing patients to tell them that you have been delayed for whatever reason can often calm a situation, particularly if it is accompanied by an apology. When staff must visit clients who are located in high-rise buildings that seem to present security risks, they should exercise special care in elevators, stairwells, and unfamiliar residences.[2]

On reaching a person's house, community staff should stand away from the door when it is being opened to them, and take time to make a risk assessment before taking up an offer to enter. If they feel at risk of harm to themselves, they should make an excuse, leave, and arrange for an alternative appointment. Risks can include alcohol or drug-abusing family or friends, or psychotic individuals. In such situations, and according to procedures that have been established, staff should immediately leave the premises. The reasons for their leaving should be reported and logged. They should not return unless escorted or until the hazard has been removed. They should also be aware of animals in the house and ask for them to be removed, prior to entering. Remember that the initial assessment is the time when you know least about the client and the environment in which they live.

On entering the patient's environment, the same precautions and safe guards can be exercised as described in Chapters 3 and 4, with adaptation to the new situation. Of particular importance here is to identify points of entry and egress. Always attempt to position yourself near a doorway or a conspicuous window. In addition to this, the community worker should be prepared to readdress the goals of their visit if the situation is not what they expected, and leave if they feel threatened or unsure. Avoid potentially perceived threats to a client or their family, and confront judiciously, never mediate in a domestic quarrel. Consideration should be given to the type of shoes and clothes that are worn by the community worker. Clothing should be appropriate, bland and do nothing to excite the patient. Shoes should not hinder movement or the staff member's ability to run. The healthcare worker should avoid wearing things that might snag or which the person may grab, such as earrings, necklaces etc. Likewise, staff should refrain from wearing things around their neck that may be used to strangle or choke, such as stethoscopes and identification badges on chains.

Animals

If there is a known problem with animals at a particular address or location, the occupants should be contacted and requested to remove or secure the animals before arrival. Some clinical procedures may provoke a reaction from an animal or pet, so it may be wise to request that it be removed or placed in a different room for the duration of the visit.[2] This might, however, provoke a negative reaction in the owner and this should be borne in mind when making the request.

Organisational factors

From an organisational point of view, there is need to ensure that there are always enough staff to cope with any foreseeable violence. Written working procedures need to specify the staff required to implement them. Discussions about staff levels and competence need to take into account issues such as:[10]

- the acceptability of lone working and the possibility of pairing staff for certain visits
- limiting the length of time staff work alone
- the need to cater for unpredictable workloads.

Above all, no staff member should be left alone in a situation where they do not feel safe, or able to manage. Staff must be provided with appropriate training in personal safety awareness and physical skills; this training must be part of an ongoing programme, and staff must be updated regularly.

The DHSS committee included the following questions in its report.[11] The first set of questions are aimed at managers and ask:

1 are your staff who visit:
   – fully trained in strategies for the prevention of violence?
   – briefed about the area where they work?
   – aware of attitudes, traits or mannerisms that can annoy clients, etc?
   – given all available information about the client from all relevant agencies?
2 have they:
   – understood the importance of previewing cases?
   – left an itinerary?
   – made plans to keep in contact with colleagues?

– the means to contact you – even when the switchboard may not be in use?
– your home telephone number (and you theirs)?
– a sound grasp of your organisation's preventive strategy?
– authority to arrange an accompanied visit, security escort or use of taxis?

3 do they:
– carry forms for reporting incidents?
– appreciate the need for this procedure?
– use them?
– know your attitude to premature termination of interviews?
– appreciate their responsibilities for their own safety?
– understand the provisions for their support by your organisation?

The second set of questions are aimed at staff:

1 have you:
– had all the relevant training about violence to staff?
– a sound grasp of your unit's safety policy for visitors?
– a clear idea about the area into which you are going?
– carefully previewed today's cases for potential for violence?
– asked to 'double up', take an escort or use a taxi if unsure?
– made appointments?
– left your itinerary and expected departure/arrival times?
– told colleagues, manager, etc about possible changes of plan?
– arranged for contact if your return is overdue?

2 do you carry:
– forms to record and report 'incidents'?
– a personal alarm or mobile phone? Does it work? Is it handy?
– a bag/briefcase, wear an outer uniform or car stickers that suggest you have money or drugs with you? Is this wise where you are going today/tonight?
– out-of-hours telephone numbers, etc to summon help?

3 can you:
– be certain your attitudes, body language, etc will not cause trouble/defuse potential problems and manage aggression?

Activity 6.1

Photocopy the home visit check list on the next pages. Place a tick next to each question you can answer in the positive and a cross against those that you do not meet. The more crosses you have, the more at risk you are in visiting patients in the community.

Home visits (example of good practice)

1 Before leaving

  1.1   Check:
      ☐   records, anything known
      ☐   route and location; be sure how and where to go
      ☐   vehicle, fuel OK

1.2   Let others know
- [ ] where you are going and how long you will be
- [ ] ring at regular intervals
- [ ] ensure car registration numbers are at base

1.3   Difficult visits
- [ ] ring in prior to and after visit

1.4   Colleagues covering your visits
- [ ] brief colleagues on difficulties

1.5   Accompanied visits
- [ ] do you have a local policy on when you request other staff to assist?
- [ ] NB some police forces will try to provide an escort where imminent danger is threatened, subject to resources available

1.6   Doubts
- [ ] if in doubt, double check address and telephone number
- [ ] check the telephone directory or ask the operator to confirm, consider ringing back to confirm
- [ ] verify information about previous treatment; ask caller to be visible at house window or door as you arrive and to leave light on/ curtains drawn back at night
- [ ] do not become a victim
- [ ] assess the situation and needs before leaving

2   En-route

2.1   Consider
- [ ] the time
- [ ] the location
- [ ] the route

2.2   Procedure
- [ ] lock car – while driving if necessary
- [ ] do not leave medical bag on view
- [ ] being followed? uneasy? uncertain?
- [ ] remain with or return to your vehicle, drive away for a short while, drive to a place of safety
- [ ] if your suspicions are confirmed, contact the police

3   On arrival

- [ ] be alert
- [ ] be aware
- [ ] be safe
- [ ] park with care, ensure you can pull straight out from parking position

If in doubt:

- [ ] do not enter premises
- [ ] seek advice
- [ ] seek assistance
- [ ] plan out action

4   Personal safety

- [ ] park in well-lit area
- [ ] do not take shortcuts
- [ ] do walk facing oncoming traffic
- [ ] do carry a torch if dark

☐ do have a personal alarm readily at hand
☐ do avoid groups of rowdy people
☐ if provided, ensure mobile phone is on and charged on return to car
☐ do have keys ready
☐ do check the interior before getting in
☐ lock the door immediately you get in
NB Minimise the risks – think ahead

5 Keeping you and your car safe
☐ lock it
☐ close the windows
☐ do not leave property in view
☐ do not leave medicines/prescription pads
☐ do not advertise doctor or nurse on call unnecessarily
☐ fit and use security locks
☐ do not leave registration documents in car

6 Equipment
☐ torch
☐ personal alarm
☐ does everything work?
☐ check batteries and carry spare

(Lincolnshire Partnership NHS Trust, 2004. *Lone Working Policy.*)[6]

References

1 Beale D, Fletche, B and Leather P. *Review of Violence to NHS Staff Working in the Community*. Nottingham: University of Nottingham; 1998.

2 NHS Security Management Service (NHS SMS). *'Not Alone' A Guide for the Better Protection of Lone Workers in the NHS*. London: NHS SMS; 2005.

3 NHS Health Development Agency. *Violence and Aggression in General Practice*. London: Department of Health; 2002.

4 Linsley P. Aggression. In: Mallick M, Hall C and Howard D. *Nursing Knowledge and Practice*. London: Ballière Tindall; 2004, pp. 245–61.

5 Royal College of Nursing. *Safer Working in the Community: a guide for NHS managers and staff on reducing the risks of violence and aggression*. London: Royal College of Nursing; 1998.

6 Lincolnshire Partnership NHS Trust. *Lone Working Policy*. Lincoln, Lincolnshire Partnership NHS Trust; 2004.

7 Mayhew C. *Occupational Violence and Prevention Strategies*. Master OHS and Environment Guide. CCH Australia, North Ryde; 2003, pp. 547–69.

8 National Audit Commission. *A Safer Place to Work: protecting NHS hospital and ambulance staff from violence and aggression*. Report by the Controller and Auditor General HC527 Session 2002–03. London: The Stationery Office; 2003.

9 Health Development Agency. *Violence and Aggression in General Practice: guidance on assessment and management*. London: Health Development Agency; 2001.

10 NHS Security Management Service. *Protecting your NHS: a professional approach to managing security in the NHS*. London: Department of Health; 2003.

11 Department of Health and Social Security (DHSS). *The Report of the DHSS Advisory Committee on Violence to Staff*. London: Department of Health and Social Security; 1988.

Chapter 7

Special considerations: gender, violence, health and healthcare

Julie Dixon, edited by Paul Linsley

Introduction

Health and healthcare are not mutually exclusive concepts and as such there is a need to examine the gendered implications of violence in relation to both health and healthcare. The seriousness of the situation is one that is gaining increasing attention, as the issue of violence against women becomes ever more apparent and the need to tackle it more urgent.

General facts and figures

In general, men tend to be more aggressive than women. In England and Wales men commit over 90% of violent crime; half of these are committed by males aged 17–24 years, and this is usually directed towards women.[1,2] Given these findings, it comes as little surprise that most women know their attacker and have some kind of association with them. Violence against women is no longer hidden, but contested within the public domain. Sex inequalities that are common in society are often reflected in the health sector.[3] Healthcare professionals often meet women who have been abused, most notably in accident and emergency departments and midwifery services.[4,5]

Violence against women is considered to be one of the most pervasive human rights violations in the world.[6] For this reason many believe that when discussing violence we need to highlight that for the most part we are talking about 'male violence' and thus it is gender based. Yet we tend to refer to violence in a gender-neutral way. Hoffman claims that:

> Gender-neutral language is used to describe a behaviour when it is assumed to be the norm.[7]

In the 18th century, English common law gave a man permission to discipline his wife and children with a stick or whip no wider than his thumb. This 'rule of thumb' prevailed in England and America until the late 19th century.[8] Such beliefs may be seen to still exist today. For example, The Edinburgh Zero Tolerance Project found that one in five young men and one in ten young women thought that violence against women was occasionally acceptable.[9]

A study by Elliot and Shannahan found that one in five people (20%) felt it was okay for a husband to hit his wife under certain circumstances, for example, infidelity, not being obedient and not having meals ready on time.[10] They concluded that the 'circumstances' were often based on role expectations, in that men judged their wives' behaviour as inappropriate and responded 'appropriately'.

The notion that our society condones and encourages violence against women is not a new phenomenon. One only needs to look at advertising to see that violence against women is considered 'normal' and/or erotic. Attitudes are further shaped and influenced through social institutions e.g. legal and educational systems, and in some ways can be said to be endemic.

Nature/nurture

The focus here is on the 'sex' hormones, however there is much research that considers other biological determinants of violence for example studies of brain lesions (*see* also Chapter 2).

For the purpose of this chapter I will use the terms testosterone (and related androgens) to refer to the male sex hormone and oestrogen and progesterone as the female sex hormones, although I acknowledge that the picture is not that simple.

The overwhelming stereotype is that testosterone is the cause of aggressive behaviour in men and that this leads to male violence. An 'average' woman has 40–60 ng testosterone per decilitre of blood plasma, and men have on average 300–1000 ng/dl.[11]

Wilbur claims that testosterone is the evolutionary 'fuck it/kill it' (FIKI) tool which is a part of the male 'appetite survival system' that has evolved as a survival instinct.[12] He further suggests that men fuse together sexual desire and violence as a means of asserting authority and control over women. A similar view is held by O'Reilly who suggested that testosterone is a biological tool to express and protect.[13]

More recently, studies have considered the role of oestrogen and progesterone in relation to female violent/criminal behaviour, more specifically the role of premenstrual stress (PMS) or premenstrual dysphoric disorder (PMDD). PMS and/or premenstrual tension (PMT) are terms widely used in western public discourse. Frank (a medical practitioner) first used it in 1931; at this time it was used to describe the monthly fluctuation of mood and behaviour experienced by women. Today it is a 'classified' mental disorder. In the *Diagnostic and Statistical Manual of Mental Disorder (DSM)* (1994), PMDD is characterised by depressed mood, irritability, increased anxiety and a lack of motivation and energy.[14] In order for a diagnosis of PMDD to be given, a woman has to experience, recurrent emotional and physical symptoms (there are over 150 listed) in the week prior to menstruation and continue for the first two days of menstruation. It has been estimated that 5–95% of women suffer (to some extent) from this disorder, suggesting that the majority of women experience (to some extent) mental illness on a regular (monthly) basis.[15] The medical profession generally believes that the hormonal fluctuations are the cause of the problem. Many women experience such changes in mood on a regular basis.

There is much controversy within the arena of mental health in terms of whether PMDD is a mental disorder or not. Regardless of this there are a number of legal cases in the UK, whereby judgment has been passed that the women involved were not held responsible for the actions on the grounds of diminished responsibility. Medical literature is confusing and limited on the possible connection between PMS and criminal behaviour.[16] Johnson identifies a woman with no previous criminal record; after a fight with her lover she drove her car at him, ramming him into a lamp post.[17] While charged with murder, the court reduced the charge to manslaughter on the grounds of diminished responsibility due to PMS.[16] This has led to concerns amongst feminists as to the implication of such biological determinism. Chesler suggests that medico-scientific discourse uses PMS within a patriarchal society to control and constrain women.[18] Reducing women to their raging hormones and negating women's experiences ('is it *that* time of month?'), can only serve to undermine women, who are viewed as being too emotionally volatile and as such should stay 'in the home!'. While there is recognition that female sex hormones fluctuate, women are not necessarily driven by them and indeed the monthly fluctuation may be the only time that women feel able to express themselves. Nonetheless women often attribute their 'symptoms' to the menses and childbirth, and these are thus central to the way women understand their feelings.[17]

Some believe that these 'problems' are socially constructed in that if women believe menstruation to be problematic they will experience it as such, a self-fulfilling prophecy.[19] Perhaps the reason why women are less violent is because their *aggressive* hormones only appear once a month; for the rest of the time it is argued that women internalise their anger in a manner befitting a 'lady'.[18] There is also concern that 'Like all medical disorders, a whole class of people with similar maladies can be stigmatised'.[16]

Interestingly, studies of male and female prisoners found that testosterone affects the behaviour of both men and women, in that testosterone levels were higher in men who had committed violent crimes; such men and women (with higher levels of testosterone) tended to violate prison rules more often. They concluded that testosterone plays an important role in male and female criminal behaviour, but that other variables such as age, social factors and other hormones also needed to be considered.[20] In a study of men who had been castrated to calm them 9 out of 16 died as a result of violent encounters, perhaps the loss of testosterone affected their ability to win, rather than their aggressive tendencies.[21] It would appear that removing testosterone does not remove violent behaviour, but may have a calming effect!

A study by Sapolksy offers a useful example in relation to the nature/nurture debate.[22] Wild spotted female hyenas in Kenya have higher levels of testosterone than their male counterparts, their genitalia are similar in appearance to males, and the females are more dominant and more aggressive. Pups were removed from their 'natural' habitat to the University of California; with the same high levels of testosterone, females found it difficult to establish dominance. The suggestion is that there is no social system to learn from.[7] So while testosterone levels correlate with increased dominance and aggression there is no causative link! Indeed this example suggests that it is the social structure and socialisation that are important factors when considering dominant/aggressive behaviours.

Testosterone levels also fluctuate in relation to external circumstances, for example testosterone levels are elevated after a fight or within highly charged sexual environments, for example, within a strip club. Studies of inner-city youths who are exposed to high levels of crime show they tend to have higher testosterone levels than, youths from the suburbs.[11] Testosterone is also considered vicarious in that those watching sport experience fluctuations in testosterone levels. Those supporting the winners see a rise, and those backing the losers see levels fall.

The cognitive effects of testosterone however are rarely studied.[23] Dabbs' *NSF* [National Service Framework] *Progress Report* considered testosterone in relation to violence and concluded that the effects of testosterone are smaller and more varied than is commonly believed, and that testosterone does not work in isolation.[23] There is a need to understand the interactions between gender and social systems in order to understand male violence; without this knowledge it will not be possible to tackle the problem.[7]

Violent and aggressive behaviour is considered to be a consequence of complex biological and environmental factors. For instance high-stress environments can contribute to high amounts of aggression, high levels of aggression can led to high levels of stress and so we have a self perpetuating 'cycle of violence'.[24]

In an attempt to provide a sociological perspective on gender and violence I have given priority to the social construction of masculinity. It has been suggested that the construction of masculinity is at the roots of male violence against women.

Feminism, masculinities and power

As with much of this chapter, concepts such as health and violence are difficult to define; the same is also true of masculinity and femininity. Masculinity/femininity are often viewed in psychological terms in that they are something internal, however there are different ways of understanding masculinity/femininity for example gendered experiences/behaviours, role expectations, relations of power and institutional practices. Many feminists believe that violence against women is a gendered issue and a product of the social construction of masculinity. Most of the research on masculinity is constructed around representations of feminism.[25] As with feminism, masculinists are not a homogenous group and there is much literature written by heterosexual/homosexual men; some support feminist views and others are anti-feminist, but many men's groups formed in the 1970s as a response to the 'second wave' of feminism. Bristow claims that this reaction masculinity is men wanting their own version of feminism.[25,26]

Nonetheless both feminism and masculinities are challenging traditional gender roles and identities and raising public awareness of the many issues surrounding sexuality and violence. This has led to the suggestion that men are having an identity crisis, being under pressure to conform to masculine stereotypes and are viewed as being oppressed:

> It has rarely occurred to men to criticize masculinity. It is their territory, they identify themselves by it. In its name they undergo all kinds of suffering and commit all kinds of atrocities, but they do not question it. They see masculinity as a law of nature. It makes them feel at ease; it is proof of their power. They do not imagine that it could be their prison. (cited in Allwood, 1998, p. 46[25])

The term 'hegemonic' masculinity is often used. Hegemonic refers to the cultural dynamic, by which a group claims and sustains a leading position.[27] These are systems of power which gives advantage to one group over another. Our common-sense ideas can be a system of hegemonic power, which we are unaware of. Such ideas are based on the characteristics of a small number of men; however large numbers of men and women are complicit in sustaining the hegemonic model.

> We come to know what it means to be a man in our culture by setting our definitions in opposition to a set of 'others' – racial minorities, sexual minorities and above all women. (Kimmel, 1994, p. 120[28])

> The hegemonies definition of manhood is a man in power, a man with power, and a man of power. (Kimmel, 1994, p. 125[28])

Traits associated with hegemonic masculinities include dominance over women, superiority complex, emotional repression, aggression.

The term *gender* refers to the economic, social, political and cultural attributes and opportunities associated with being male and female. In most societies, men and women differ in the activities they undertake, in access and control of resources and in the participation in decision making. In most societies women as a group have less access than men to resources, opportunities and decision making.[29]

According to Lerner gender is the:

> costume, a mask, a straitjacket in which men and women dance their unequal dance. (Lerner, 1996, p. 238[30]).

Thus gender is not fixed and is changing, it is complex and shapes our intra- and interrelationships, performing masculinity in today's society can and does lead to male violence. Violence against women is an integral part of a patriarchal culture and it serves to keep men in a dominant position.

Increasing numbers of media articles emerged in the 1980s suggesting that men have changed after 10 years of feminism. This has led to the belief that men were losing their identity. Alia has suggested that the 'new man' has emerged from a 20-year process.[31] Becoming initially good househusbands and fathers, being bored with this they moved onto 'feminised man' to 'infantilised man', women could not resist mothering them and men no longer had to take responsibility. Alia does however question how 'new' a concept this is,[31] and indeed a third of the men studied had not changed at all and many young people asked did not want the change and wanted a return to traditional role expectation.[25] Such information is having an impact for some in terms of gender relations. Violence against women is one example of the unequal power relations that exist between men and women in society. The 'new woman' of the late 19th century was viewed by many as a fictional caricature of the Victorian feminist;[32] maybe the 'new man' is a fictional caricature of masculinists.

Hearn argues that masculinity is either seen in psychological/internal terms or socially as a set of practices, which reflects masculinity as if it is something that resides inside of men.[33] He recommends that we need to consider masculinities and avoid generalised assumptions about masculinity, which can be used to explain men's behaviour historically and culturally, suggesting a look at what men actually do, think or feel – the material realities of the way men act in the social world.

Gender conformity brings about benefits, if one wants to please ones parents or peers, for example. Discourse theory is about power within relationships, and as such is something that can be challenged.[34] Masculinity is not something that one fits into, but is constantly being constructed and negotiated with every interaction; some match stereotypes (conformity) others offer resistance. Masculinity and power are institutional. The complex interactions of the origins of western hegemonic masculinities are important. Their roots have many discursive influences within society, for example medical, educational, religious knowledge and practices. For instance, Tomaszewski gives examples of male violence (e.g. pulling hair, lifting up skirts etc) of girls in primary schools in Australia.[2] The 'system' did little to stop the violence, with the notion that 'boys will be boys'. The message is clear that if one is a boy, it is okay to behave in this way. Boys did not understand that what they were doing might be considered offensive or even illegal.

One female teacher claimed that:

> If we don't intervene we are allowing primary schools to be training grounds where the links between masculinity and violence become cemented. (cited by Tomaszewski, 2005, p. 336[2])

Some girls had worked out that if they got a boyfriend he would protect her; the role of men then is to either perpetrate violence or protect from male violence. Please note however that these concepts are not exclusive as many protectors become perpetrators (and vice versa). Most women who experience violence know the perpetrator, and more often than not is in, or has been in, an intimate relationship with him.

Looking at the social construction of masculinity highlights the many discursive influences that shape our understanding of men, women and their behaviour. Men and women are no longer driven or passive respondents to their *sexual* hormones, but can be viewed as victims of discursive influences. There is also the need to consider material conditions.[35] All of these issues appear to absolve the individual of responsibility for his/her behaviour.

Question

Is gender something we perform?

Violence and abuse

Violence against women refers to a wide range of physical, sexual, emotional and financial abuse. The more common forms of abuse towards women are as follows:

- *sexual abuse*: forcing or encouraging someone to take part in sexual behaviour in any way that makes them uncomfortable

- *sexual harassment*: any objectionable, unwanted, or unwelcome attention to a person because of his or her sex
- *domestic violence*
- *rape*
- *pornography*: while gaining increasing legitimacy, there remains a large amount of pornographic material in which violence towards women is portrayed. This diminishes the worth and civil status of women and gives the social message that this type of abuse is sanctioned.

Other forms of violence to women include:

- *Female genitalia mutilation (FGM)*: this comprises all procedures involving partial or total removal of the external female genitalia or other injury to the female genital organs whether for cultural, religious or other non-therapeutic reasons
- *dowry deaths*: in certain cultures a dowry is paid to the future husband by the family of the bride. The dowry often consists of money, merchandise, or gold that is displayed when the couple is married and is determined by the perceived value of the husband's hand in marriage. Women are being mistreated if they have insufficient monies. If the bride's family cannot provide more for the in-laws they will kill her so that he may keep the dowry he had already collected and then is able to remarry
- *female infanticide*: is the intentional killing of baby girls due to the preference for male babies and from the low value associated with the birth of females. It is closely linked to the phenomena of sex-selective abortion, which targets female fetuses almost exclusively, and neglect of girl children.

Domestic violence

Often described as the 'hidden crime' as it is under-reported and often happens in the home, despite this domestic violence statistics suggest that one in four women are affected and it accounts for a quarter of all violent crimes in England and Wales.[36]

Domestic violence has been defined as:

> any violence between current and former partners in an intimate relationship, wherever and whenever the violence occurs. The violence may include physical, sexual, emotional, financial abuse.[37]

Furthermore, children are often witness and subjected to this type of abuse and there would seem to be a correlation between domestic violence and the mental, physical and sexual abuse of children.[38]

A large-scale study of primary care and domestic violence (*see* Box 7.1) found that 41% of the women studied had (at some point in their lives) experienced physical violence from a partner or former partner; 74% experienced controlling behaviour by a partner; 46% had been threatened; 21% had had injuries; 15% had reported violence, 29% of these stated this led to miscarriage during pregnancy.[39] Domestic violence accounts for 25% of all recorded violent crimes and two women are killed each week by their partner or former partner.[40] In the UK 45% of female murder victims were killed by their partner or former partner,

---

Box 7.1 Domestic violence

Domestic violence includes:

- *physical violence*: biting, bruising, burning, choking/strangling, hitting, kicking, knifing, murder, punching, scalding, scratching, slapping, sleep deprivation, starving
- *sexual abuse/assault*: forced sex – anal/vaginal/oral, urinating on, sexual assault using objects, forced tying up, enforced prostitution, being forced to mimic pornography/take part in pornography
- *psychological abuse*: criticism, verbal abuse, isolation from family and friends/work, humiliation and degradation, extreme jealousy and possessiveness, financial deprivation, being made to think they are going mad, threats, destroying personal belongings, being forced to do menial/trivial tasks.

---

while the comparable figure for men is 8%.[35] Such statistics suggest that men are more abusive than women and gives evidence for the 'need to provide dedicated services to protect women and their children from domestic violence'.[40] This is not to say that women are not abusive and/or violent.

Women who experience violence are significantly more likely to report health problems and have long-lasting consequences to health and individual well-being.[41,42] Partner abuse occurs in all types of relationships (homosexual and heterosexual), and male violence against women is a problem in public health terms.[43] Domestic violence is rarely found to be a one-off event, and attacks tend to become more frequent and increasingly severe over time.[44]

Domestic violence and abusive relationships affect the health of women in terms of:[45]

- physical injuries
- chronic problems e.g. irritable bowel syndrome (IBS), headaches
- increased unwanted pregnancies, terminations and lower birth weights
- higher rates of sexually transmitted infections (STIs) (including HIV)
- higher rates of depression, anxiety, post-traumatic stress disorder (PTSD), self-harm and suicide.

Healthcare practitioners may be reluctant to acknowledge violence or to seek evidence of it for a number of reasons.[45] These include:

- fear of taking the lid off something which will get out of control
- fear of not knowing what to do next
- fear of causing offence
- belief that this is not the province of the NHS
- personal identification with abuse either as a victim or perpetrator.

Indicators that may signal domestic violence include:[45]

- does the woman make frequent appointments for vague complaints or symptoms?

- are appointments often missed?
- are there injuries that seem inconsistent with the explanations of accidental causation (such as falls or walking into doors etc), and are these injuries to the face, neck, chest, breast or abdomen?
- is there evidence of multiple injuries at different stages of healing?
- does the woman try to minimise the extent of her injuries?
- does the woman appear frightened, excessively anxious or distressed?
- does the partner or other family member always accompany the woman when she attends a consultation?
- does the partner appear aggressive and overly dominant? And is the patient passive and afraid?

Screening for domestic violence is difficult and should be done by those who have been trained in such matters. However, raising concerns about a woman who may have experienced domestic violence should not be avoided. Sometimes reluctance may be a reflection of particular beliefs or prejudices about domestic violence. It may be believed, for example that:[43]

- domestic violence is not a serious issues, or that it is essentially a private matter between partners
- women provoke violence and 'ask for it'
- some women deliberately choose violent men
- such matters are better dealt with by other agencies other than health, for example, by social services or the police.

People who have experienced domestic violence may similarly be reluctant to disclose what has happened to them. Reasons for reluctance include:[44]

- fear of an unsympathetic response
- fear of reprisals and serious escalation of violence from their partner if they get outsiders involved
- shame and embarrassment over what has happened to them
- fear that their children will be taken into care
- lack of awareness that help might be obtained from health professionals
- fear of the police or other authorities being contacted and for some black and ethnic minority women – fear of deportation.

It is therefore vital that healthcare professionals are sensitive to clues and indications that might suggest domestic violence. While women may be reluctant to disclose what is happening to them, often they are hoping that someone will realise that something is wrong and ask them about it.

Principles of conduct

- Ensure that the safety of the women (and of any dependent children) is the paramount consideration.
- Treat people with respect and dignity at all times; listen to what they are saying and do not be judgemental; establish empathy and trust.

- Seek to empower people to make informed decisions and choices about their lives, and do not try to make decisions on their behalf.
- Respect confidentiality and privacy, and recognise the real dangers that may be created if this is breached.
- Recognise the skills and contributions that other agencies are able to make, and co-operate with them.
- Ensure that you do not place yourself or your colleagues at risk in a potentially violent situation.

A review of screening for domestic violence in health services found that there was insufficient evidence for screening programmes, but that services should aim to identify and support women.[46] Taket *et al.* however differentiate between the use of screening (standardised questions) and routine inquiry, and recommends that questions about domestic violence become a part of routine inquiry, thus uncovering hidden cases, changing perceptions of acceptability to violence in relationships, challenging attitudes towards violence, reducing stigma and above all keeping women safe from experiencing domestic violence.[43] Without intervention the abuse continues; abuse is not only cyclical but tends to be progressive, in that the violence tends to escalate in terms of frequency and severity.[46] Health professionals are in the right place to identify domestic violence, but this cannot happen without sufficient training and increased knowledge of advice and support services.

Activity 7.1

Prepare a list of local resources that may be helpful when assisting someone who has been subjected to domestic violence. This might include, support groups, local refuges, crisis lines and the local authority emergency housing service.

Women's health

The World Health Organization (WHO) defined health as:[47]

> a state of complete physical, mental and social well-being and not merely the absence of disease or infirmity.

This suggests that health relates to the social and physical environments, and is a consequence of relationships of individuals and groups within social structures.

Experience of child sexual, physical and emotional abuse, all forms of domestic violence and sexual assault/rape (both inside and outside the home), are common among women and are a significant factor in the development of mental ill-health (and its many manifestations) and physical ill-health.[37]

There is a strong link between childhood sexual abuse and deliberate self-harm; such violence towards self is considered to be a manifestation of women's distress. The experience of abuse often erodes women's self-esteem making them vulnerable to mental health problems. Fifty per cent or more of women within the mental health system are survivors of violence and abuse; percentages are higher in secure settings.[46] Busfield claims that 89% of women with a diagnosis of borderline personality disorder are survivors of prolonged and severe abuse (notably sexual abuse).[35] It has been argued that these women are experiencing post-traumatic stress disorders and advocate trauma-based therapies are advocated.[43]

Children's health

Children growing up with domestic violence are 30–60% more likely to experience abuse and have higher rates of:

- sleep problems
- poor school performance
- emotional detachment
- stammering
- suicide attempts
- aggressive and disruptive behaviour.

Moreover children learn to accept violence as a way of life, and often repeat the patterns in adulthood.[43]

'Malestreaming' services

The term gender malestreaming came into use after the Beijing 'Platform for Action' in 1995 UN International Conference for Women. Malestreaming is about issues surrounding gender equality for men and women, an integral part of the work of organisations, including issues of employment law through to governance, service delivery and outcome. The term is now used within healthcare, and services are becoming increasingly aware of the need to target men's and women's health issues within policy development.

Most healthcare professionals work in a 'malestream' context in so far as senior managers and policy makers, regardless of gender, can perceive violence against women as a social and legal issue, and many have to be cajoled to take seriously the potential role of health services in supporting women who wish to disclose abuse.[48]

Many healthcare staff will be experiencing similar abuse in their own intimate relationships. However employers' and government interest lies in the violence that exist against staff, for instance the *NHS Zero Tolerance Zone*.[49]

Violence in the healthcare setting

It is not only patients that are abusive to staff, but abusive practice is also widely documented, for instance, D'Oliveria *et al.* discuss four types of violent abuse by doctors and nurses: neglect, verbal, physical and sexual abuse.[50] These categories are similar to those in personal relationships. They identify that such abuse occurs and relates to poor and ineffective healthcare services. They claim that this abuse is learnt in training and reinforced in the practice setting. Organisations have a duty of care to their employees (Health and Safety at Work Act 1974 (*see* Chapter 8)). They also have a duty of care to those who use the service.

Question

Should healthcare professionals ask patients if they are being abused? Debate this question with colleagues.

A national audit found that one in three in patients had experienced violence or threatening behaviour, clinical staff 41% and nurses 81%.[51] Violence has not solely been directed from patients to staff, but from staff to staff and from staff to patients. Gender differences are marked, with women reporting higher levels of sexual harassment as a form of threat. A study of 586 nurses in seven states in the United States reported that sexual harassment was included in the definition of workplace violence by 78% of the nurses.[52] Such differences perhaps are embedded in the gendering of particular occupations. Nurses, for instance, are more likely to be women, and, as noted early in the book, nursing receives a higher proportion of assaults and intimidation at work than other healthcare occupations.

Training and development

The Department of Health in the *Mainstreaming Gender and Women's Mental Health. Implementation Guidance,* recommends the following in terms of dealing with violence in the healthcare setting:[40]

- identify signs and symptoms of violence and abuse
- develop skills in assessment, ensuring sensitivity to asking questions about violence and abuse
- develop understanding of the aspects of confidentiality
- provide safe environments for disclosure
- provide information on available support.

Meeting the needs of women, health professionals need to challenge issues of power and abuse in their own lives at work and in society. Offering training for service users will not be effective if staff themselves are being abused and are afraid to do anything about it. Unless attitudes towards violence against women change, the situation is likely to get worse. Health professionals need the support to deal with their own experiences of violence in order to help those that they care for. Issues of gender and gender-sensitive approaches need to be included within all healthcare training programmes and not seen as a separate issue. However, training is not enough, working conditions and staffing levels need to be considered so that staff can give the time, privacy and dignity to service users. Effective discipline is needed for staff who abuse service users, whistle-blowers need to be supported.

Conclusion

This chapter has been about gender, violence, health and healthcare. While much has been done to highlight male violence against women, much needs to be done to 'treat' and deal with the problem. Many feminists have argued that violence is a gender issue and is a product of the social construction of masculinities.

Perhaps the thought of dealing with the political and cultural aspects of violence in society is too big an issue to be addressed within the healthcare setting. Many continue to deny the problem, suggesting it exists outside in 'deprived' communities, despite the evidence that violence varies very little by geography, race and ethnicity.[41]

Gender and violence is not solely a health and healthcare issue, but has social and economic implications for all government departments and services as well as for those who use the service.

National and local policies need to develop along with research. Documents like *Mainstreaming Gender and Women's Mental Health* offer a good place to start,[40] but their implementation can only be successful if people start to challenge destructive gendered beliefs.

Not all violence is the same! Our brains mediate all behaviour, and brain development is a product of biology and environmental influences. All such issues need to be taken into account when considering the 'treatment' of violence. There is not one single solution. Power relations are interactive and reciprocal. There is a need for knowledge about the ways in which men and women interpret, perceive and express their gender. Our beliefs determine our choices and behaviour. Whatever the form of violence, it needs to be stopped; challenge of traditional gender definitions needs to occur.

References

1 Mulholland C. *Men and Violence: do you have a problem with that?* www.netdoctor. co.uk/menshealth/feature/men_and_violence.htm (accessed 20 December 2005).

2 Tomaszewski I (2005) *Preventing Adult Sexual Assault: violence, gender and power and the role of education* http://216.239.59.104/search?q=cache:_wi3ErpqcscJ:www. aic.gov.au/publications/pr (accessed 20 December 2005).

3 Austin J. *Violence and Aggression: managing the risk to NHS Staff.* Health Service Manager Briefing No. 66. Surrey: Corner; 2001.

4 British Medical Association (BMA). *Domestic Violence: a health care issue.* London: British Medical Association; 1998.

5 Royal College of Midwives. *Domestic Abuse in Pregnancy.* Position paper. London: Royal College of Midwives; 1998.

6 Bond J and Phillips R. *Violence against women as a human rights violation: international responses.* In: Renzett IC, Edleson J and Bergen R (eds). *Sourcebook on Violence against Women.* London. Sage; 2001.

7 Hoffman E. *Violence, Gender and Health.* www.zmag.org/ZSustainers/Zdaily/ 2000–09/08hoffman.htm (accessed 20 December 2005).

8 No Safe Place: violence against women. *Origins of Violence Against Women.* www. pbs.org/kued/nosafeplace/studyg/origins.html (accessed 20 December 2005).

9 Coward R. Number crunching: do young people condone domestic violence? *The Guardian.* 16 February, 1998.

10 Elliot PR and Shannahan R. *Domestic Violence in Australia.* Office of the Status of Women, Department of Prime Minister and Cabinet; 1988.

11 Sullivan A (2005) The he hormone. *The New York Times Magazine.* www.photius. com/feimnocracy/testosterone.

12 Wilbur K (1996) *A Brief History of Everything.* www.dickmanagement.com/ch03. htm

13 O'Reilly S. Testosterone – the fuck it/kill it biohazard. http://www.dickmanagement. com/ch03.htm (accessed 20 December 2005).
14 American Psychiatric Association (1994) *Diagnostic and Statistical Manual of Mental Disorder (DSM)* (4e) APA, Washington.
15 Ussher J. *Women's Madness – Misogyny or Mental Illness?* London: Harvester Wheatsheaf; 1991.
16 Easteal P. Women and crime: premenstrual issues. *Trends & Issues. Crime and Criminal Justice.* 1991; **31**: 1–9.
17 Johnson S and Buszewicz M. Prevalence of mental disorder in the community. In: Abel K, Buszewicz M, Davison S *et al* (eds). *Planning Community Mental Health Services for Women.* London: Routledge; 1996.
18 Chesler P. *Women and Madness.* NewYork: Doubleday 1972.
19 Cochrane R. Women and depression. In: Niven C and Carrol D (eds). *The Health Psychology of Women.* Berkshire: Harwood Academic Publishers; 1993. In: Mallick M, Hall C and Howard D (eds). *Nursing Knowledge and Practice: foundations for decision making* (2e). London: Baillière Tindall; 2004.
20 Dabbs J and Hargrove M. *Testosterone linked to Violence in Female Inmates.* www. scienceblog.com/community/older/1997/A/199700216.html (accessed 20 December 2005).
21 Sterling FA. *Myths of Gender, Biological Theories about Women and Men.* New York: Basic Books; 1992.
22 Sapolksy R. *The Trouble with Testosterone and other Essays on the Human Predicament.* London: Simon and Schuster; 1997.
23 Dabbs J. *Hormonal Influences in Nonviolent Dominance.* NSF Progress Report 09/ 9608/99. www2.gsu.edu/~psyjmd/NSF96–99
24 Cox C (2001) Biology and Aggression http://serendip.brynmawr.edu/biology/ b103/f01/web2/cox
25 Allwood G. *French Feminisms: gender and violence in contemporary theory.* London: UCL Press; 1998.
26 Bristow J (1990). In: G Allwood. *French Feminisms: Gender and violence in contemporary theory.* London: UCL Press; 1998.
27 Gramsci A. *Selections from Political Writings. 1921–26.* London: Lawrence and Wishart; 1971.
28 Kimmel MS. Masculinity as Homophobia: fear, shame and silence in the construction of gender identity. In: Brod H and Kaufman H (eds.) *Theorising Masculinities.* London: Sage Publications; 1994.
29 Beijing Platform of Action (1995) Cited in: Department of Health. *Mainstreaming Gender and Women's Mental Health. Implementation Guidance.* London: Department of Health; 2003.
30 Lerner G. *The Creation of Patriarchy Oxford.* Oxford University Press; 1996.
31 Alia J (1991). In: G Allwood. *French Feminisms: Gender and violence in contemporary theory.* London: UCL Press; 1998.
32 Reynolds K and Humble N. *Victorian Heroines: representations of femininity in 19th century literature and art.* Hertfordshire: Harvester Wheatsheaf; 1993.
33 Hearn G. Cited in: Macan Ghaill M. *The Making of Men. Masculinities, sexualities and schooling.* Buckingham: Open University Press; 1994.
34 Foucault M. *Discipline and Punish: the birth of the prison.* New York: Vintage; 1979.
35 Busfield J. *Men, Women and Madness. Understanding gender and mental disorder.* London: MacMillan Press Ltd; 1996.
36 Spencer A. Speak out. *NHS Magazine.* **February 2005**: 22–3.
37 Stevens L. A Practical Approach to Gender-Based Violence: a programme guide for health care providers and managers: Developed by the UN Population Fund. *International Journal of Gynecology and Obstetrics.* 2002; Suppl. 1. **78**: 111–17.

38 Hammer J. Women and policing in Britain. In: Hammer J, Radford J and Stanko E (eds). *Women, Policing and Male Violence*. London: Routledge; 1989.
39 Richardson J, Coid J, Petruckevitch C *et al.* Identifying Domestic Violence: A Cross-Sectional Study in Primary Care. *British Medical Journal*. 2002; **324**: 274.
40 Department of Health. *Mainstreaming Gender and Women's Mental Health*. Implementation Guidance. London: Department of Health; 2003.
41 Commonwealth Fund, Department of Health DoH. *Violence and Abuse*. www. cmwf.org/programs/women/ksc_whsurvey99_fact4_332.asp.
42 Royal College of Nursing. *Position Paper on Domestic Violence*. London: Royal College of Nursing; 2000.
43 Taket A, Nurse J, Smith K *et al.* Routinely asking women about domestic violence in health settings. *British Medical Journal*. 2003; **327**: 673–6.
44 Royal College of Nursing. *Domestic violence: guidance for nurses*. London: Royal College of Nursing; 2004.
45 Department of Health. *Domestic Violence: a resource manual for health care professionals*. London. NHS Executive; 2000.
46 Ramsey J, Richardson J, Carter YH *et al. Should Health Professionals Screen Women for Domestic Violence?* Systematic review. *British Medical Journal*. 2002; **325**: 314.
47 Klein R. Sickening relationships: gender-based violence, women's health and the role of informal third parties. *Journal of Social and Personal Relationships*. 2004; **21**: 149–65
48 McKie L. Review Article. Gender, violence and health care: implications for research, policy and practice. *Sociology of Health and Illness*. 2003; **25**: 120–31.
49 Department of Health (1999) *NHS Zero Tolerance Zone: we don't have to take this*. Resource Pack. London: HMSO; 1999. www.nhs.uk/zerotolerance/downloads/index-htm
50 D'Oliveria A, Diniz SG and Schraiber LB. Violence against women in health-care institutions – an emerging problem. *Lancet*. 2002; **359**: 1681–5.
51 BBC News World Edition. *Violence Widespread in NHS Units*. Monday 23, 2005. BBCNews/uk/Violence widespread in NHS Units .
52 Occupational Safety and Health Administration (OSHA) *Guidelines for Preventing Workplace Violence for Health Care and Social Service Workers*. Washington, DC: Occupational Safety and Health Administration; 1998.

Useful contact numbers

Women's Aid Federation of England
England's national charity for women and children experiencing physical, sexual or emotional abuse in their homes. 24-hour domestic violence helpline.
Tel: +44 (0)8457 023 468
www.womensaid.org.uk

Scottish Women's Aid
Tel: +44 (0)131 475 2372
www.scottishwomensaid.co.uk

Welsh Women's Aid
Tel: +44 (0)29 2039 0874

Northern Ireland Women's Aid Federation
Tel: +44 (0)2890 331818
www.niwaf.org

Refuge
24-hour UK-wide domestic violence crisis line
Tel: +44 (0)8705 995 443

Kiran – Asian Women's Aid
Advice, support, refuge and outreach help for Asian women and children
Tel: +44 (0)20 8558 1986

Southall Black Sisters
Information and advice for black and Asian women on domestic violence and related issues.
Tel: +44 (0)20 8571 9595

NSPCC
Child protection helpline for anyone in England, Wales or Northern Ireland concerned about the safety of a child. Asian language service also available.
Tel: +44 (0)808 800 5000
www.nspcc.org.uk

Everyman Project
Counselling, support and advice for men who are violent or concerned about their violence, and anyone affected by that violence
Tel: +44 (0)20 7737 6747

Home Office
Loves Me Not – Leaflet on domestic violence
www.homeoffice.gov.uk

Chapter 8

Special considerations: legal issues

Introduction

The management of violence and aggression makes explicit the need to have an understanding of legal principles and law[1,2] This will aid staff in the decision-making process and lead to greater confidence when taking charge of a challenging situation (*see* Figure 8.1). The examples given in the following chapter are based on the law pertaining to England and Wales; this is similar to the law in Scotland and other countries across the European Community.

Legislation

Consideration must be given over to the different sources of law and the system by which the legal process works. Legislation and the law that comes from it define the behaviour by which a society is to operate through powers of enforcement and sanction. A *statute* is an Act of Parliament that sets out the law in a formal document. Each Act of Parliament follows a detailed procedure of debate and voting in the House of Commons and the House of Lords. Statutes form a body of law that set out in detail how individuals must act. In this way a statute is the formal laying down of a rule or rules of conduct to be observed by those to whom the statute is expressly or by implication made applicable. Legislation also comes from membership of the European Community, which requires its member states to implement community law through their own Acts of Parliament. Directives encompass a variety of issues, including statements on the hours people should work and the manner in which they should be treated as part of their employment.

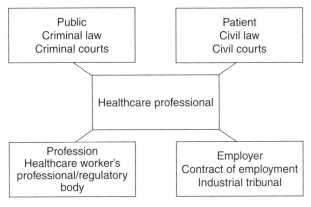

Figure 8.1   Arenas of accountability. Adapted from Dimond (1992).[5]

Criminal law

Criminal law is founded on statutes. Anyone breaking this type of law is likely to be charged formally by the police and tried in a court of law before a judge and jury, for example theft. The criminal law system is designed to allow the accused to dispute allegations before a representative section of the community. It is the task of the jury to decide *beyond reasonable doubt* whether or not the person is guilty of the charge for which he or she stands accused. Penalties for digression are intended as a punishment although there may be some compensation. The types of penalties include binding over – ordering a criminal to obey the law, under the threat of suffering penalties for the crime if convicted of additional crimes, fines and in some cases jail.

The seriousness of harm caused by violence is usually considered in terms of physical injuries sustained. Legally, this is reflected in the relative severity of charges that are associated with criminal violence, which can be levelled for a variety of contact offences, ranging from the slightest degree of unwanted physical contact right up to murder, with other charges that are applicable to different degrees of physical harm along this continuum. However, it should be acknowledged that threats, verbal abuse and physical assault can also result in emotional damage being sustained by targets, which can in some instances exceed the degree of physical harm inflicted. Indeed, the potentially serious degree of harm that can be inflicted without physical contact being made has now been recognised by law, with successful prosecutions for grievous bodily harm being brought against stalkers.

Case or common law

Case law is made by judges and forms the greatest proportion of the law of the country. Where no legislation exists to determine law on a particular subject, case law will be used. Case law is based on precedent: previous decisions will normally be applied to similar cases unless the judge can identify features which distinguish the current case from the previous one. In deciding a case, the two sides will present their views of the facts and will direct the judge to relevant precedents. If there is no jury, the judge decides which version of the facts is to be believed and, based on those facts and precedents, decides what the law is, and how it is to be applied in the particular case. In applying case law, the judge will look at the relevant case report and extract what he or she believes to be the principle behind the decision of the judge who decided the original case. Although a judge will be guided by the statement of reasons and other comments given in an earlier judgement (particularly if it is a judgement from a senior court such as the House of Lords), the abstraction they decide upon is not necessarily what the original judge would have chosen. This is permissible because under British law, judges do not make the law by formulating and stating it but by applying it to cases coming before them. If there is a jury, they will be informed of the relevant law by the judge, and will then reach a decision based on the facts of the case as they see them.

Judges can escape the bounds of precedent by:[3]

- distinguishing the present case by finding some facts which make it different from the previous case
- deciding that the principle of the previous case is too obscure to be used
- declaring that the previous case is in conflict with a fundamental principle of law (i.e. it was wrong)
- finding that the previous case was decided in ignorance of a relevant case or statute
- finding that a new statute over-rules the previous decision
- finding that there are several similar cases with conflicting decisions at the same level.

This gives judges significant flexibility in applying the law in particular circumstances to reach what they believe to be a just decision. The courts are all bound by higher courts, which can over-rule a decision at a lower level. Any change in case law would affect the current case and future cases, but not any previous cases that had been decided. The House of Lords has asserted its right not to be bound by a previous decision. This provides an important way of allowing an unjust decision to be changed without relying on Parliament to change the law by statute.

Civil law

Civil law is designed to resolve differences between individuals. As a consequence, civil law encompasses a wider range of issues than does criminal law, including negligence, employment, divorce, child care, libel, defamation and any other matter that is not criminal in nature. A side must prove its case on the *balance of possibilities* in order to secure an outcome.

Prosecution

A target of assault has the right to report the incident to the police, or their employer could do so on their behalf. It is a decision for the police and the *Crown Prosecution Service* (CPS) whether or not they take action against an individual for the assault, wherever the assault occurs. Influencing factors in the CPS and the police deciding whether to proceed with prosecution include the severity of the assault, the mental health state of the assailant and the context of the assault. If the injuries sustained are serious and result in the healthcare worker taking time off work to recover physically or psychologically, it is possible to make an application to the *Criminal Injuries Compensation Board*, which can make a separate award of compensation for injuries received as a result of a violent attack, without the necessity for a criminal prosecution.

One of the most important factors in the decision whether to pursue prosecution is the desired outcome. A major issue in the interface between mental healthcare and the criminal justice agencies is the question of what are the purpose and benefits of prosecution. Is it for the benefit of the patient (identifying unmet needs), the benefit of the target (retribution) or of those who are thought to be at risk of further assault (protection of the public)? An arbitrary policy may lead to significant defects in its implementation.[4]

Legal forums

Disputes that need to be resolved within the legal system will be heard in public, except in cases where a vulnerable person is involved such as in child abuse or mental health cases, to safeguard anonymity.

Industrial tribunals deal with disputes relating to employment, including bullying and harassment. The tribunal has power to hear employment cases and make rulings, which include the power to order reinstatement or a payment of compensation if a finding of unfair dismissal or discrimination is made.

An *inquest* is another legal forum, the purpose of which is to investigate the circumstances of a death that may not have been natural or expected. A coroner directs the hearing and can put questions directly to witnesses. A jury sits and listen to the evidence and returns a verdict in relation to the circumstances of the death.

Where incidents are considered to be of national concern then a *public enquiry* can be called for. A report is published after the enquiry has ended and recommendations made to remedy the problems leading to the crisis. The public inquiry into the death of David 'Rocky' Bennett, following restraint resulted in a number of changes to the management of disturbed patients, in particular how a person was to be held.[5]

Negligence

When a procedure such as physical restraint goes wrong and involves injury to a person then the possibility of an action of negligence must always be considered. In order for liability for an injury to be established, the following conditions must apply:[5]

- there must be a duty of care owed by one person to another
- the person failed to observe this duty of care by falling below the standard of care expected
- the injury caused must arise directly from the duty of care that has been broken.

In English law, the test of this standard of care which is employed in medical negligence claims is known as the *Bolam Test*, which states that treatment should be considered lawful if it is administered in accordance with the opinion of a responsible body of professional opinion (*see* Box 8.1).[6] While the existence of an opposite point of view is not sufficient to support a claim of negligence, the court may choose to disregard the precedence of the opinion of a responsible body of professional opinion if it believes that such opinion and practice falls below the standard that can be reasonably expected under the circumstances.

Box 8.1   Standard of care

When you get a situation which involves the use of some special skill or competence, then the test as to whether there has been negligence or not is

---

> ... the standard of the ordinary skilled man exercising and professing to have that special skill. If a surgeon failed to measure up in that respect (clinical judgement or otherwise) he had been negligent and should be so adjudged.
>
> (*Whitehouse* v. *Jordon*, 1981 A11ER267)

Given the above, it is possible for a patient to sue an individual practitioner or their employer for compensation in respect of injury sustained through the negligent application of restraint. In defence, it would be necessary for the practitioner or his/her employer to demonstrate that:

1 the potential risk of injury had been recognised, and appropriate training to designated competencies had been sought or provided
2 the risk of harm to the patient or others if restraint was not applied was greater than the potential risk of injury during restraint[7,8]
3 a responsible body of professional opinion held that the actions of the practitioners in attempting to restrain the injured person were reasonable.

It may also be possible for a patient who receives injury as a result of assault by a fellow patient to sue the provider of care for damages. In defence, the provider would have to demonstrate that:

1 the assault was not reasonably foreseeable, or
2 the acts or omissions of members of staff providing care in that environment did not fall below a reasonable standard, or, if the care provided did fall below such a standard, that this did not materially contribute to the patient's risk of being assaulted.

Self-defence

Staff are legally entitled to use a measure of self-protection if they fear an attack from a patient or other while on duty. They can do so by using what is termed 'reasonable force'. This concept is complex, and it can only be determined in any particular instance in a court of law. However, it has been defined by Dimond as:[5]

> the force used should be no more than was necessary to accomplish the object for which it is allowed (so retaliation, revenge and punishment are not permitted) and secondly, the reaction must be in proportion to the harm which is threatened in both degree and duration.

The measure of defence must therefore be in proportion to the threat or attack itself: it would be reasonable for a healthcare worker to push a patient who made to hit them, but it would not be reasonable for the member of staff to do this if the patient was shouting abuse. This suggests that if a client can usually be dealt with by non-physical means, the use of physical force or restraint would constitute an assault.[8]

The potential target has a duty to retreat and escape, and it is only where no opportunity to escape is available that self-defence is likely to be considered legitimate.[9] Since this excuse is a 'private defence', it is not restricted to the defence of one's own person, but can be extended to the protection or others (e.g. patients, other staff, or visitors), and can be used to justify defending oneself (or others) from assault by an 'innocent aggressor' (such as a patient who is mentally ill).[10] Since a potential target can make 'reasonable' efforts to prevent harm, it is not necessary to wait for a blow to be struck before taking action.

This provision also enables a member of staff to use reasonable force in an attempt to prevent a patient committing an assault or any other criminal offence (although for very minor offences the use of force is unlikely to be considered reasonable). Attempts of suicide however would not meet these criteria, as that act itself is not a criminal offence. However, restraint of a person who was in the process of committing an act of self-harm or suicide would generally be permissible using 'lawful excuse' that the member of staff owed a duty of care to the individual concerned.

The use of force or the restriction of liberty must, even where lawful excuse exists, meet the criteria of reasonableness. In using such measures the individual's actions will be judged with regard to the facts of the situation as the individual perceived them to be at the time of their action, even if, in hindsight, this judgement was wrong or the grounds for his/her judgement are considered unreasonable.[11]

Restraint of a patient or person

Any restriction on the liberty or autonomy of a person may constitute a criminal offence unless lawful excuse for such actions can be offered. Paterson *et al.* describe the potential criminal charges that could possibly result, and the potential defences to such charges.[9] Potential charges include:

False imprisonment

This is defined as:

> an act of the defendant which directly and intentionally or negligently causes the confinement of the plaintiff within an area delimited by the defendant.

Confinement in this context effectively means a situation where an individual is prevented from leaving a particular place (e.g. hospital or its grounds, a room, or other particular area). The restriction of liberty must effectively be 'total', in that the patient would be likely to injure himself or herself if they attempted to leave, or it would be considered unreasonable to expect the patient to leave the situation.

Assault and battery

Assault is defined in English law as:[12]

> any act of the defendant which directly and either intentionally or negligently causes the plaintiff immediately to apprehend a contact with the person.

The requirement of immediacy in the crime of assault is generally understood to mean that the target must perceive the threat as one which can be carried out 'there and then' by the defendant. There is no need for any physical contact between the defendant and the target. The emphasis is on what the target thought was about to happen. So even if the defendant meant his threat as a joke, an assault is nevertheless committed if the target is sufficiently frightened

Battery is defined as:[13]

> any act of the defendant which directly and intentionally or negligently causes some physical contact with the plaintiff without the plaintiff's consent.

Again such charges may potentially be defended against with reference to the concepts of 'lawful excuse' and 'reasonable force', however comparability would have to be decided in each case before a verdict could be reached.

Breach of the peace

This is a situation where:[14]

> harm is done or likely to be done to a person or in his presence, to his property: or harm is feared through an affray, riot, assault or other disturbance.

A person in this situation has both the duty and the right in common law to use reasonable force to stop the person concerned from breaching the peace, which would apply to attempts made by the healthcare worker (or even a fellow patient) to prevent a threatened or actual breach of the peace committed by a patient whose words or behaviour fulfil the criteria above.[14]

Sex Discrimination Act 1975 and the Race Relations Act 1976

Both these Acts deal in part with verbal abuse and harassment in specific contexts and are enforced by the Equal Opportunities Commission and the Commission for Racial Equality respectively.

Public Order Act 1986

The Public Order Act 1986 covers the use of threatening, abusive or insulting behaviour that is likely to cause harassment, alarm or distress, as well as physical assault, and is enforced by the police. The Act itself can only be applied after an offence has been committed, and cannot be used to require the taking of preventative measures. One implication of this is while police forces expend considerable effort in promoting prevention of such crime, they have no powers to enforce such measures.

Protection from Harassment Act 1997

The Protection from Harassment Act introduced in 1997 provides protection against abuse through two criminal offences: that of *criminal harassment*, and the more serious *offence involving fear of violence*. Harassment is defined as behaviour which would be regarded as harassment by a 'reasonable person'. A perpetrator is guilty of the offence of causing fear of violence when they know or ought to know that their course of conduct will cause the other fear (on at least two occasions). This offence is seen as useful in allowing the courts to take action *before* serious psychological or physical harm occurs.[15]

Health and safety legislation

Employers have a duty of care for the health and safety of their employees and this duty is incorporated into health and safety legislation. The overall requirement to protect the health and safety of employees is contained in the Health and Safety and Welfare at Work Act 1974. The duties covered within this legislation are subject to the test of being 'reasonably practicable'. This means that only if the cost of taking the necessary preventative measures is grossly disproportionate to the risk is there justification for taking no action. The requirements on employers, under the health and safety legislation, have been summarised by the Health Services Advisory Committee and the Royal College of Nursing.[16,17] They are as follows:

The Health and Safety and Welfare at Work Act 1974

Employers must:

- protect the health and safety of their employees
- protect the health and safety of others who might be affected by the way they go about their work.

The Management of Health and Safety at Work Regulations 1992

Employers must:

- assess all risks to the health and safety of their employees
- identify the precautions needed
- make arrangements for the effective management of precautions
- appoint competent people to advise them on health and safety matters
- provide information and training to their employees.

Reporting of Injuries, Diseases and Dangerous Occurrences Regulations (RIDDOR 95)

Employers must:

- report all cases in which employees have suffered death or major injury or have been off work for three days or more following an assault that has resulted in physical injury including 'acts of non-consensual physical violence'. This however does not apply to non-workers and absence from work due to causes that are not physical, e.g. illness resulting from verbal abuse, or psychological conditions arising from physical assault.

The above duties must be applied to all aspects of the working environment where hazards could lead to harm for those at work and to others who might be affected by what happens in the workplace. It is clear that violence and aggression are an occupational health and safety hazard which is covered by the legislation, and one that must be acted upon. Failure to comply with such legislation could lead to enforcement action by the Health and Safety Executive. The range of enforcement starts from the issue of improvement notices through to criminal prosecution and fines.

The obligations of the employee

While it is the responsibility of the employing organisation to provide safe systems of work, individuals also have a responsibility to follow safe working practices. *Vicarious liability* is the term used in law to illustrate this principle.[17] An employer is vicariously liable for the acts or omissions of their employee in the course of their employment (in other words that the employee acted within policy and procedure). To avoid vicarious liability, an employer must demonstrate either that the employee was not negligent in that the employee was reasonably careful or that the employee was acting in his own right rather than on the employer's business (acting outside of policy and procedure). There are a variety of situations in which a party may be charged with vicarious liability. Employers can face a number of situations involving vicarious liability issues, including sexual harassment of one employee by another, discriminatory behaviour by an employee against fellow employees or customers, or any other action in which one of their employees personally causes harm, even if that employee acts against the policies of the employer.

The *Employment Rights Act 1996*, Section 44, provides employment protection in connection with health and safety. It prevents an employer from taking action such as dismissing or disciplining an employee who leaves their place of work because of danger, which they believe to be 'serious and imminent', and which they could not be reasonably expected to prevent. This includes taking any appropriate steps to protect themselves or others from the danger. For example, a community nurse is protected from any action by their employer if they leave a client's home because of abuse or violence from the client or the relative.

The Public Interest Disclosure Act 1998

This Act protects whistle-blowers from victimisation and dismissal when they speak out, but their concerns must be genuine and must have been raised (unless there are very good reasons for not doing so) internally or with a specified person. It reflects public concern about the difficulties for workers to speak out when they believe something is seriously wrong in their workplace.

In order to be protected, the disclosure has to show one or more of the following has occurred:[18]

- a criminal act
- a failure to comply with legal obligation (including negligence, breach of contract, including contract of employment, and breach of administrative law)
- a miscarriage of justice
- danger to health and safety
- damage to the environment
- an attempt to cover up any of these.

It is sufficient for the worker to have a reasonable belief that their information is correct; this means that the worker will not have to prove their disclosure is accurate, but they will need to demonstrate that they acted in good faith.

The *Safety Representatives and Safety Committees Regulations* (1997) and *The Health and Safety (Consultation with Employees) Regulations* (1996), state that employers must inform and consult with employees on matters relating to their health and safety (including possible violence and aggression), and that employee representatives may make representations to their employer on matters affecting their health and safety.

Zero tolerance

The Department of Health launched the NHS Zero Tolerance campaign in October 1999.[19] to inform the public that (a) aggression, violence and threatening behaviour will not be tolerated by staff working in the health service, and (b) get the message over to all staff that violence and intimidation towards them are unacceptable and are being tackled. In addition to this, the guidance aims to balance staff protection with the duty to provide services, and states that care will be denied to clients who abuse staff. Verbal abuse, vandalism, drug and alcohol abuse, are all identified as grounds for refusing treatment. Understandably, a number of criteria must be met before treatment can be withdrawn. The government says care is not to be denied to clients with severe mental health problems or other conditions that clinicians think leave the client incapable of taking responsibility for their actions.

The appropriateness of refusing/withdrawing treatment turns on the effect of the behaviour displayed by the person, for instance, where violent or abusive behaviour might:[19]

- prejudice any benefit from the care
- prejudice the safety of someone giving the care
- lead the employee to believe that he/she is unable to undertake his/her duties
- result in property damage by the client or through containment
- prejudice the safety of other clients.

When care must be provided to violent or aggressive patients, procedures might include the administration of medication, physical intervention, or the attendance of security personnel and/or involvement of the police.

The guidance is driven not just by health and safety requirements and the duty of care owned by employers but also by the *Human Rights Act 1998*. This act seeks above all others to protect the dignity and feelings of employees from 'inhuman' or degrading' treatment on the part of the employee (Article 3). In addition to this, the campaign has been backed by new prosecution procedures for both staff and service users.

Mental Capacity Act 2005

The Mental Capacity Act provides a statutory frame work to protect vulnerable people, carers and professionals when the capacity of an individual to make decisions regarding their safety and wellbeing is called in to question. The Act starts from the fundamental point that a person has capacity, and that all practical steps must be taken to help the person make a decision. Of particularly concern is the individual's ability to exercise choice and provide consent.

The Act sets out a clear test for assessing whether a person lacks capacity to take a particular decision at a particular time. It provides a checklist of factors that decision makers must work through in deciding what is in a person's best interests. The Act makes it clear that a person can provide care or treatment for someone who lacks capacity, without incurring legal liability. Restraint is only permitted if the person using it reasonably believes that it is necessary and proportionate to prevent harm.

Crime and Disorder Act 1998

Finally, with the passing of the Crime and Disorder Act 1998, local authorities and police, in co-operation with other bodies such as the NHS trusts and health authorities, are legally required to develop and implement crime and disorder strategies. Some trusts are actively involved with local crime prevention groups to share information, advice and intelligence on particular issues which might influence how best to manage difficult situations.

References

1 Paterson B and Tringham C. Legal and ethical issues in the management of aggression and violence. In: Turnbull J and Paterson B (eds). *Aggression and Violence: approaches to effective management*. Basingstoke: Macmillan; 1999.
2 Young PA. *Law and Professional Conduct in Nursing* (2e). Harrow: Scutari Press; 1994.
3 Rawls S. *A Theory of Justice*. Oxford: Oxford University Press; 1992.
4 Coyne A. Should patients who assault staff be prosecuted? *Journal of Psychiatric and Mental Health Nursing*. 2002; **9**: 139–45.
5 Dimond B. *Legal Aspects of Nursing* (2e). London: Prentice Hall; 1992.
6 Home Office and the Department of Health. *Mentally Disordered Offenders: Inter-Agency working*. London: HMSO; 1995.
7 Reed J. Risk assessment and clinical risk management: the lessons from recent inquires. *British Journal of Psychiatry*. 1997; **32**: 4–7.
8 Davies RW. Controlled aggression. *Nursing Times*. 1996; **2**: 18–9.
9 Paterson B, Tringham C, McComish A *et al*. Managing violence and aggression: a legal perspective on the use of force. *Psychiatric Care*. 1997; **15**: 128–31.
10 Brazier M. *Clark and Lansdell on Torts* (16e) London: Sweet and Maxwell; 1989.

11 Lyon C. *Legal Issues Arising from the Care, Control and Safety of Children with Learning Disabilities who Present Severe Challenging Behaviour*. London: Mental Health Foundation; 1994.

12 Temple CM. Managing physical assault in a healthcare setting. *Rehabilitation Nursing*. 1994; **19**: 281–6.

13 Litterell KH and Litterell SH. Current understanding of violence and aggression: assessment and treatment. *Journal of Psychosocial Nursing and Mental Health Services*. 1998; **36**: 18–24.

14 Trade Union Congress. *Violent Times: preventing violence at work*. London: Trade Union Congress; 1999.

15 Martin A. The case for self defence. *Health and Social Service Journal*. 1990; **11**: 697.

16 Smith JC and Hogan B. *Criminal Law* (6e). London: Butterworth; 1988.

17 Department of Health. *Domestic Violence: a resource manual for health care professionals*. London: Department for Health; 2000.

18 Health and Safety Advisory Committee. *Violence and Aggression to Staff in Health Services: guidance on assessment and management*. Sudbury: HSE Books; 1997.

19 Care and Health. *Zero Tolerance – drawing the line in health and social care*. www.careandhealth.com (accessed 21 December 2005).

Index